Nursing Research: Qualitative Methods

Publishing Director: David Culverwell
Acquisitions Editor: Richard Weimer
Production Editor/Text Design: Barbara Werner
Art Director: Don Sellers, AMI
Assistant Art Director: Bernard Vervin
Manufacturing Director: John A. Komsa

Indexer: Leah Kramer
Typesetting: Action Comp Co., Inc., Baltimore, Maryland
Printing: R. R. Donnelley & Sons Co., Harrisonburg, Virginia

NURSING RESEARCH

QUALITATIVE METHODS

ROSEMARIE RIZZO PARSE, RN, PhD

Professor of Nursing
Hunter College Graduate Nursing Program
New York, New York

A. BARBARA COYNE, RN, PhD

Director, The Dwelling Place Center for Health
Pittsburgh, Pennsylvania

MARY JANE SMITH, RN, PhD

Professor of Nursing
West Virginia University
Morgantown, West Virginia

BRADY COMMUNICATIONS COMPANY
A Prentice-Hall Publishing Company
Bowie, Maryland

Library of Congress Cataloging in Publication Data

Parse, Rosemarie Rizzo.
  Nursing research

  Bibliography: p.
  Includes index.
  1. Nursing—Research—Methodology. I. Coyne, A. Barbara, 1929–   . II.
Smith, Mary Jane, 1938–   . III. Title. [DNLM: 1. Nursing. 2. Research.
WY 20.5 P266n]
RT81.5.P36   1985   610.73'072   84-24312
ISBN 0-89303-724-9

Prentice-Hall of Australia, Pty., Ltd., *Sydney*
Prentice-Hall Canada, Inc., Scarborough, *Ontario*
Prentice-Hall Hispanoamericana, S.A., *Mexico*
Prentice-Hall of India Private Limited, *New Delhi*
Prentice-Hall International (UK) Limited, *London*
Prentice-Hall of Japan, Inc., *Tokyo*
Prentice-Hall of Southeast Asia Pte. Ltd., *Singapore*
Editora Prentice-Hall Do Brasil LTDA., *Rio de Janeiro*
Whitehall Books, Limited, Petone, *New Zealand*

Printed in the United States of America

85 86 87 88 89 90 91 92 93 94 95   1 2 3 4 5 6 7 8 9 10

CONTRIBUTORS

Nancy J. Andre, MSN
Veterans' Administration Medical Center
Aspinwall, Pennsylvania

Lisabeth K. Kraynie, MSN
Sewickley Valley Hospital
Sewickley, Pennsylvania

Sharan J. Magan, RN, PhD
Veterans Administration Medical Center
Highland Drive
Pittsburgh, Pennsylvania

Marlaine C. Smith, MSN
Pennsylvania State University
Pittsburgh, Pennsylvania

Carol Z. Weiner, MSN
Gannett Health Center
Cornell University
Ithaca, New York

Writing a book is an adventure. To begin with, it is a toy and an amusement ... then it becomes a master, then it becomes a tyrant. The last phase is that just as you are about to be reconciled to your servitude, you kill the monster and fling him to the public.

WINSTON SPENCER CHURCHILL

CONTENTS

LIST OF TABLES

PREFACE

The purpose of research in nursing is to guide the evolution of nursing science through the enhancement and verification of theoretical perspectives, which guide practice and further research. The purpose of this work is fourfold: 1) to present the basic elements of selected qualitative methods; 2) to demonstrate the use of these selected methods from one nursing perspective, the theory of Man*-Living-Health; 3) to set forth criteria for the critical appraisal of qualitative studies; and 4) to provide a demonstration of the use of the critique elements. The methods chosen for presentation are from established research traditions in the social sciences and existential phenomenology and are used from a nursing perspective. Borrowing a method and adapting it to the nursing perspective alters the pure form of the method as defined by the discipline of origin. It is through borrowing methods in this way that emerging disciplines, such as nursing, carve out their own research traditions. In borrowing qualitative methods from other disciplines, the presentations in this book modify the grounded theory view of Glaser and Strauss (1967), which specifies that qualitative research generates theory grounded in empirical observation.

The specific modifications reflected in the studies are that phenomena are conceptualized within a particular nursing perspective and findings interpreted in light of that perspective. The five research studies presented here are written only to demonstrate the method and therefore do not include nursing implications.

This book is intended primarily for graduate students at both the masters and doctoral levels who may be critiquing and implementing qualitative research studies. It is also useful for baccalaureate students who are seeking an understanding of the qualitative research process, and will be helpful to faculty in guiding the qualitative research process. The organizational pattern of the methods chapters (III, VI, and VIII) is designed around the five basic ele-

---

*In this work, the term man refers to *homo sapiens*. Man is a generic term that includes both Men and Women.

ments of research: 1) identifying the phenomenon; 2) structuring the study; 3) gathering the data; 4) analyzing the data; and 5) describing the findings. The structure for the demonstration chapters (IV, V, VII, IX and X) follows a similar pattern using these primary aspects: 1) purpose; 2) research question; 3) phenomenon; 4) conceptual framework or researcher's perspective; 5) sample; 6) protection of subjects' rights; 7) data gathering; 8) data analysis; and 9) discussion of findings.

This work is offered as a contribution in the continuous development of research traditions in the discipline of nursing.

I

NURSING RESEARCH TRADITIONS
QUANTITATIVE AND QUALITATIVE
APPROACHES

Research traditions in a discipline emerge from the paradigms of that discipline. A paradigm, according to Thomas Kuhn, (1970) is a world view; a way of looking at a field of study. The paradigm contains the basic beliefs about the phenomena of concern in the discipline. For nursing, the phenomena of concern are Man and Health. Two paradigms in the discipline of nursing can be distinguished by their inherent beliefs about Man and Health. These paradigms may be referred to as the Man-environment-totality paradigm and the Man-environment-simultaneity paradigm. In the *totality paradigm*, Man is considered a bio-psycho-social spiritual being reacting and adapting to the environment. Man is an organism whose behavior can be measured and predicted as well as changed through management of the environment. Health is considered a state of well-being that can be identified and altered by health professionals according to social expectations. In the *simultaneity paradigm*, Man is considered a synergistic being in open, mutual, simultaneous interchange with the environment. Man chooses from options and bears responsibility for the outcome of choices. Man cocreates patterns of relating with the environment; and both Man and environment are recognized through these patterns. Health is viewed as a non-linear entity, a process of becoming experienced by the individual. It is Man's negentropic unfolding (Parse 1981).

These two paradigms, the totality and the simultaneity, reflect different beliefs about Man and Health and thus require different methods of inquiry in their research traditions. Research traditions are peculiar to a discipline and flow directly from the beliefs of the paradigms within that discipline.

Nursing has no unique research traditions (Donaldson and Crowley 1977, Gorenberg 1983). Scholars are presently developing these traditions. In the emergence of a scientific discipline, borrowing research methods that most closely relate to the paradigmatic perspective is appropriate and necessary. This use of borrowed methods from other disciplines leads to the carving out of unique research traditions. In nursing's emergence as a science, it has borrowed research methods from other disciplines. Nursing research that focuses on testing conceptual systems from the totality paradigm reflects the beliefs about Man and health within that paradigm. For these research studies, quantitative methods have been borrowed from the natural sciences to study Man as an organism adapting to the environment while striving for a state of well-being. The quantitative methods include experimental, quasi-experimental, descriptive correlational, ex post facto, and exploratory designs.

For research studies focusing on phenomena from the simultaneity paradigm, research methods have been borrowed from the human sciences. The qualitative methods, in which Man's lived experiences are studied, focus on description as their primary outcome and explicitly express a value for the thoughts, perceptions, and feelings of subjects about lived experiences. As more nursing systems evolve from the simultaneity paradigm, more nursing research studies will be conducted using the qualitative methods.

Gorenberg (1983) specifies a need for the development of nursing's research traditions with use of qualitative methods for research studies. Little has been written in nursing literature about the qualitative methods and very few qualitative studies have been published. Watson (1981) called for a new research tradition that can provide nursing with the scientific freedom to work within the unique domain of human experience. Oiler (1982), Omery (1983), and Knaack (1984) presented the phenomenological method and Ragucci (1972) proposed the ethnographic method as options for nursing research.

The qualitative methods, to be addressed in this text, include the social science descriptive method, which includes the case study and the exploratory study; the phenomenological method; and the ethnographic method.

There are major differences between the quantitative and qualitative approaches to research, relating to the fundamental meanings of quantitative and qualitative and to the paradigmatic perspectives described above. Quantitative refers to the attribution of numbers to measure variables. The measured characteristics in quantitative research should be reliable and valid indicators of the variables being studied and the numerical scores should be objective, precise, and unbiased. Quantitative data are processed through statistical analyses and elicit numerical comparisons and inferences.

Qualitative research identifies the characteristics and the significance of human experiences as described by subjects and interpreted by the researcher at various levels of abstraction. In qualitative research the researcher's interpretations are *intersubjective*, that is, given the researcher's frame of reference, another person can come to a similar interpretation. Qualitative data are processed through the creative abstractions of the researcher as the subjects' descriptions are studied to uncover the meaning of human experiences.

The differences between the quantitative and qualitative approaches to research related to paradigmatic perspectives can be divided into three major characteristics. They are: 1) Conceptual—the nature of the phenomenon, 2) Methodological—the handling of data and 3) Interpretive—the expected outcomes. The nature of the phenomenon refers to its paradigmatic origin. The fundamental belief about Man's nature as atomistic or synergistic will be reflected in the way the research phenomenon is identified for inquiry. The focus of inquiry is on either Man's collective attributes or Man's lived experience. The handling of data refers to collection and analysis procedures. This must be consistent with the nature of the phenomenon being studied. For example, numerical comparisons are appropriate for research studies guided by the totality paradigm but not appropriate for analyzing descriptions of lived experiences studied from the simultaneity paradigm. Expected outcomes refer to the results of the study in either making predictions about tested hypotheses or generating hypothetical propositions. Table 1 shows the differences according to these characteristics.

The qualitative approach offers the researcher the opportunity to study the emergence of patterns in the whole configuration of Man's lived experiences. It is an approach in which the researcher explicitly participates in uncovering the meaning of these experiences as humanly lived.

A unique and controversial feature of the qualitative method is the nature of the researcher's participation in data collection and analysis. In quantitative research this is referred to as *bias*. Qualitative research takes into account the researcher's frame of reference (paradigm) and makes this frame of reference explicitly part of the research report (Bodgan and Taylor 1975). The researcher's participation is called the *research-researcher dialectic*, and is a relation-

TABLE 1   MAJOR DIFFERENCES OF RESEARCH APPROACHES

	QUALITATIVE	QUANTITATIVE
CONCEPTUAL Phenomenon	1. Emerges from the simultaneity paradigm. 2. Reflects a study of Man's lived experiences in nonmeasurable terms.	1. Emerges from the totality paradigm. 2. Reflects a study of Man's attributes in measurable terms.
METHODOLOGICAL Data Handling	1. Gathers data through participant observation, interview, and retrospective description. 2. Analyzes data by identifying and synthesizing themes and common elements from descriptions by subjects.	1. Gathers data through physiological, psychological, and sociological measures. 2. Analyzes data through numerical comparisons and statistical inferences.
INTERPRETIVE Expected Outcomes	1. Describes lived experiences. 2. Generates hypothetical propositions through logical abstraction.	1. Predicts relationships. 2. Tests and validates hypotheses with a given statistical probability.

ship which emerges between the researcher and the focus of research as the researcher questions the phenomenon described. Although the researcher is said to hold personal views in abeyance, these views show themselves in several ways in the research process. The frame of reference is evident in the choice of the phenomenon to be studied, in the way the research question is presented, in the way the data are collected and analyzed, and in the way the results are interpreted. A primary goal of qualitative research is the generation of theory. It begins with the particular frame of reference of the researcher and descriptions of the phenomenon by subjects, and, through analysis, propositions are derived which create and enhance theories.

In qualitative research, descriptions from participant observation, structured and unstructured interviews, and written and oral retrospective accounts are studied for themes. These themes are stated in the language of the researcher, a shift in discourse significant because it moves the description of the meaning of the researched phenomenon from the subject's language to the language of science. This shift is a necessary step in theory enhancement. Pelto and Pelto (1981) make this distinction quite clear in discussing their idea of the general "domain of methodology" in scientific research. They say:

> Methodology refers to the structure of procedures and transformational rules whereby the scientist shifts information up and down the ladder of abstraction. (pp. 2-3)

According to Pelto and Pelto, the "structure of procedures" includes the conceptual framework and belief system of the researcher. It is through this conceptual framework and belief system that the shifts in levels of abstraction occur. The researcher is responsible for enhancing, enlarging, or otherwise changing the theoretical body of knowledge in the particular discipline. The transformational shifts in knowledge throughout this work are consistent with the simultaneity view in the discipline of nursing.

There are three qualitative methods presented in this book. These were chosen because they represent the recognized methods of qualitative analysis from three established disciplines, existential phenomenology, sociology, and anthropology. Within this range of disciplines there is methodological consistency. A brief description of the three methods follows.

PHENOMENOLOGICAL METHOD

This method is directed toward uncovering the meaning of a phenomenon as humanly experienced. It is a human science method which takes into account Man's participative experience with a situation. Subjects are asked to describe experiences. The researcher studies these descriptions and moves through a series of operations to a final definition of the lived experience under study. The operations for analysis differ somewhat, depending on the particular phenomenological procedure chosen by the researcher. All analytic operations, however, require the researcher to dwell with the subjects' descriptions in quiet contemplation. *Dwelling with* is profound thinking carried out through the processes of intuiting, analyzing, and describing. Through these processes, the researcher, in studying each of the descriptions, uncovers the meaning of the lived experience for each subject. The meaning surfaces as themes, or common elements, are identified and synthesized into a *structural definition* of the lived experience, which is the hypothetical proposition generated from the phenomenological study. Conclusions are then drawn relative to the research question studied.

ETHNOGRAPHIC METHOD

The ethnographic method is an open, unstructured way of looking at a phenomenon as it unfolds in everyday life, and is an appropriate method in studies related to uncovering the meaning of experiences while they are being lived. The focus is to come to know a phenomenon through the perspective of the group studied. The design includes order, system, and consistency through the processes of observation, clarification, and verification. The data collection techniques are 1) participant observation, and 2) ethnographic interview, both structured and informal.

The major vehicle for data collection in this method is the researcher, who lives the participant observation in a personal way. The procedure for data collection begins with revealing the intent of the study to the subject group. For example, one might be interested in the lived experience of fear as related to health and select Three Mile Island residents as one group of subjects to study. After reconnaissance, the researcher would take up residence in the community and tell the subject group that the general intent of the study is to learn what it is like to live in a situation after a nuclear leak. The intent of an ethnographic study may change in light of information that surfaces in the lived situation. The openness of the ethnographic method allows for shifts in intent as the ethnographer remains open to the unfolding meaning of the lived experiences of the phenomenon. The data collection procedure is primarily the ethnographic record, which consists of field notes and personal diaries gathered through participant observation and ethnographic inquiry. Data are analyzed and hypotheses proposed.

DESCRIPTIVE METHOD

This method describes the phenomenon in the context of a situation. Studies using the descriptive method begin with an explicit perspective with clearly asked questions and specific objectives. The data collection vehicles may be any one or all of the following: 1) questionnaire, 2) personal interview, and 3) observation. The procedure for data recording and analysis is specific. Information is gathered through various structured or unstructured questions. The same questions and observations are given or made with each subject if more than one subject is used. The subjects' descriptions are analyzed from the explicit perspective determined in the conceptual

TABLE 2   MAJOR DIFFERENCES OF THREE QUALITATIVE METHODS

	PHENOMENOLOGICAL	ETHNOGRAPHIC	DESCRIPTIVE
CONCEPTUAL Origin	Existentialism Phenomenology	Social Science Anthropology	Social Science
METHODO-LOGICAL Structure	Data are structured by subjects' descriptions and researcher's interpretation of the descriptions	Data are structured by the lived experience of the group and the researcher's interpretation of the experience	Data are structured by the research objectives which arise from the conceptual framework
Data Collection	Interview; Written description	Participant observation; Interview	Interview; Questionnaire
	Quality of data depends on the subjects' written and verbal skills	Quality of data depends on the researcher's lived experience with the group	Quality of data depends on the knowledge and skill of the researcher
Data Analysis	Researcher intuits, analyzes and describes the subjects' descriptions of the phenomenon	Researcher observes, clarifies, and verifies with the group living the experience of the phenomenon	Researcher collects, analyzes, and interprets data related to the research question

framework. Hypotheses are generated from the analysis and synthesis of data.

The qualitative research methods are very closely related, but have several differences in the conceptual and methodological dimensions. (See Table 2.)

The value of the qualitative method is gaining recognition and, over the next two decades, will enhance those nursing theories emerging from the simultaneity paradigm.

II

Man-Living-Health
A Man-Environment
Simultaneity Paradigm*

Research methods are chosen in light of the nature of the phenomenon being studied, the paradigm from which the phenomenon arises, and the frame of reference of the researcher. As noted in Chapter I, the qualitative methods are methods of choice when the point of inquiry is drawn from the simultaneity paradigm and its frameworks and theories. The theory of Man-Living-Health evolves from the simultaneity paradigm; thus inquiry related to it logically points to use of the qualitative methods. This chapter presents the assumptions, concepts, and principles of Man-Living-Health as a frame of reference for the qualitative studies reported in this text.

Man is a synergistic being, more than and different from the sum of parts, who is recognized through patterns of relating. Man is an open being who coexists with the universe and whose negentropic unfolding is in mutual and simultaneous interrelationship with environment. Man freely chooses among options and is responsible for choices.

Health is a process of becoming uniquely lived by each individual. It is Man's lived experience, a non-linear entity that cannot be qualified by terms such as good, bad, more, or less. It is not Man adapting or coping. Unitary Man's health is a synthesis of values, a

---

*This chapter expands ideas set forth in *Man-Living-Health: A Theory of Nursing*, by Rosemarie Rizzo Parse. (New York: John Wiley & Sons, 1981).

way of living. It is not the opposite of disease or a state that man has, but rather a continuously changing process that man cocreates.

It is from these general beliefs that the theory of Man-Living-Health emerges. The unity of Man-Living-Health is the focus of the nursing theory. Therefore, there is no reference to Man as the sum of biological, social, psychological, and spiritual attributes. This does not mean that these attributes are negated, but rather that they are viewed within the context of Man's wholeness, as shown through profiles and qualities.

Man-Living-Health is a geneologically generated theory whose assumptions emerge from a combination of Rogers's principles and four building blocks with the tenets and concepts of existential phenomenological thought (Parse, 1981). This combination created the synthesis of the nine assumptions underpinning the theory of Man-Living-Health (Parse, 1981) which have been further synthesized into the following three assumptions:

1. Man-Living-Health is freely choosing personal meaning in situations in the intersubjective process of relating value priorities.

2. Man-Living-Health is cocreating rhythmical patterns of relating in open interchange with the environment.

3. Man-Living-Health is cotranscending multidimensionally with the unfolding possibles.

There are three major themes that emerge from these philosophical assumptions. They are: Meaning, Rhythmicity, and Transcendence. These each lead to a principle of Man-Living-Health.

MEANING

According to Dilthey (1961) meaning is what expressions express and understanding understands. An expression is meaningful to the extent that it points beyond itself. Meaning arises from Man's interrelationship with the world. It refers to both ultimate meaning and the meaning moments of everyday life. Ultimate meaning is Man's conceptualization of purpose in life. Meaning moments of everyday life surface as Man confronts each moment of living. Ultimate meaning and meaning moments change through the living of new experiences. Each everyday experience stretches the boundaries of the meaning moments beyond what is, and thus sheds new light on ultimate meaning.

Imaging is the process of shaping personal knowledge. It is the creating of personal reality explicitly and tacitly all at once. The imaging (or picturing) of the world, events, ideas, and people happens in the context of valuing. The valuing process occurs simultaneously and shows an individual's cherished beliefs. Languaging is the way one represents the structure of personal reality through speech and motion, thus confirming valued images all at once. With each everyday experience, then, Man structures a personal reality reflecting new meanings incarnated through the *languaging* of *imaging* and *valuing.*

With the capacity to image and choose reality from the many levels of the universe, Man structures meaning multidimensionally. The way a person is in a situation is cocreated by a personal view and the context of the situation. The valued images are shared with others through languaging. Languaging confirms the meaning given to a situation. Thus surfaces the principle:

> Structuring meaning multidimensionally is cocreating reality through the languaging of valuing and imaging. The essential concepts of this principle are imaging, valuing and languaging. (Parse, 1981, p. 42)

RHYTHMICITY

Rhythmicity, the second theme from the assumptions of Man-Living-Health is revealed as Man and environment move toward greater diversity. Rhythmical patterns are cocreated in the Man-environment interrelationship and are paradoxes lived all at once. In every situation there is a timing and flowing process, which is lived simultaneously. Timing refers to the cadence, and flowing to the continuity evident as the changing beats become more complex. The flow of rhythms is shifted as individuals become more diverse. The shifting of rhythms surfaces in the connecting-separating process as meaning moments are stretched by new lights shed on an event.

Connecting-separating is the rhythmical process of distancing and relating, that is, moving toward one direction and away from others. *Revealing-concealing* is the rhythmical process of showing and not showing the self to self and others. Since one cannot reveal all there is of one's self to another, even what is known contains elements of the unknown, just as the unknown contains elements of the known. Man is always unfolding mystery. *Enabling-limiting* is a rhythmical process recognized as one chooses a particular direction which by its nature limits other directions. To chose one way means to give up other ways. There are an infinite number of possibilities in a particular choice; also an infinite number of limitations. Living rhythmical patterns is Man's way of coconstituting with the universe. Thus surfaces the principle:

> Cocreating rhythmical patterns of relating is living the paradoxical unity of revealing-concealing, enabling-limiting while connecting-separating. The essential concepts are revealing-concealing, enabling-limiting, and connecting-separating. (Parse 1981, p. 50)

TRANSCENDENCE

The third theme, Transcendence, is the process of reaching beyond self toward the not-yet. Man is coconstituting the actuals while simultaneously cotranscending with possibles. The possibles arise from the multidimensional experiences and the contexts of situations, and are opportunities from which alternatives are chosen. Possibles become actuals. New actuals create other possibles and in this way Man powers original transforming. What is actual is so for only one time and one place. What is and will be as it appears now, is the meaning moment that is stretched in the shifting of rhythms to the not-yet.

Transcendence is powered through originating in transforming. Powering is the pushing-resisting force of human existence recognized in the affirming of self in light of non-being. Being confronts non-being as one risks losing self. One's way of being is cocreated in connection with particular people, ideas and things, and as these connections are distanced one's way of being changes. In distancing from familiar connections, one confronts the risk of non-being, losing the self that has lived a certain history with these connections. Confronting the risk of non-being creates unrest and excitement all at once as one pushes-resists in an effort to create new connections while severing important familiar ones. Being, then, confronts non-being in the pushing-resisting of powering. Through this ever present interhuman paradoxical process Man powers transcendence.

Originating is generation of unique ways of living. This means that uniqueness surfaces in Man's continual interrogation of relationships and connections with people and projects. Although these kinds of connections are not unusual experiences, the way in which the connections are lived demonstrates the distinction which is uniqueness. To distinguish oneself in this way is to choose a unique way of living the paradoxical unity of conformity-nonconformity and certainty-uncertainty. *Conformity-nonconformity* surfaces in human encounters as individuals seek to be like others, yet at the same time not like others. *Certainty-uncertainty* surfaces in human encounters as individuals make concrete and clear choices in situations, yet simultaneously live the ambiguity of the unknown outcomes. Transcending these paradoxes in day to day encounters is originating.

Transforming is the changing of change. Change itself is a continuous process in the Man-Environment interrelationship. The transformation happens in the presence of a discovery of unique possibles as they unfold in the struggle to integrate the unfamiliar with the familiar. In this process of transforming, a person experiences struggling and leaping beyond in continuous movement toward greater diversity. The transforming unfolds in the shift of view experienced when new light is shed on a familiar situation. Thus surfaces the principle:

> Cotranscending with the possibles is powering unique ways of originating in the process of transforming. The essential concepts of this principle are powering, originating and transforming (Parse, 1981, p. 55).

These are the principles of the theory of Man-Living-Health:

1. Structuring meaning multidimensionally is cocreating reality through the languaging of valuing and imaging.
2. Cocreating rhythmical patterns of relating is living the paradoxical unity of revealing-concealing and enabling-limiting while connecting-separating.
3. Cotranscending with the possibles is powering unique ways of originating in the process of transforming.

Man participates in creating health by choosing the imaged values in multidimensional experiences that become Man's way of relating with the world. The relating is through rhythmical patterns of revealing-concealing, enabling-limiting and connecting-separating, which are lived as Man struggles in the processes of creating images, prizing values, and languaging symbols. These rhythmical processes guide Man's personal transformation through the paradoxes of living. Man-Living-Health then, is structuring meaning multidimensionally in cocreating rhythmical patterns of relating while cotranscending with the possibles.

III

THE PHENOMENOLOGICAL METHOD

The phenomenological method as a method of inquiry first appeared in the writings of philosopher Franz Brentano in the last half of the 19th century (Spiegelberg, 1976). It was further developed by Brentano's student, Edmund Husserl, and later refined by Martin Heidegger (1962). Heidegger's 20th century works brought together ideas from Husserl and Soren Kierkegaard, a 19th century existential philosopher, to create the philosophical science of existential phenomenology. The phenomenological movement was expanded by German and French philosophers in the first quarter of the 20th century. Gabriel Marcel (1956), Jean Paul Sartre (1966) and Maurice Merleau-Ponty (1974) are the pre-eminent French philosophers whose works were significant in forwarding the phenomenological movement. The French participation in the movement brought greater specificity to the meaning of existential phenomenology as a philosophy and, with this, greater diversity of thought.

The phenomenologists cannot be placed in one school or category; the diversity of philosophical thought is too great. However, they are in agreement on the method of inquiry.

PURPOSE

The phenomenological method seeks to uncover the meaning of humanly experienced phenomena through the analysis of subjects' descriptions. Knowledge about experience is expanded by allowing a phenomenon to show itself without application of the predictive prescriptions of the quantitative methodologies. The phenomenological method explicitly takes into account the human being's participation with a situation by using descriptions written or orally presented by the subjects as the raw data. It is through the analysis of the descriptions that the nature of a phenomenon is revealed and the meaning of the experience for the subject understood. And it is the major task of phenomenology to elucidate the essences of the phenomenon under investigation. This includes not only the phenomenon in itself but also the context of the situation in which it manifests itself. Phenomenology is particularly appropriate for the sciences in which Man's humanness and connection with the world are the point of inquiry. Phenomenology is a rigorous method of inquiry that requires knowledge and fine-honed skills. The researcher using this method for the first time requires a mentor who can be observed implementing the method, not merely talking about it (Spiegelberg, p. 645). In implementing the phenomenological method one must "proceed with the greatest care. For the phenomenological method is not foolproof. And plenty of fools have rushed in where neither angels nor conscientious phenomenologists have set foot. . . . There is no substitute for constant checking and rechecking. . . ." (Spiegelberg, p. 645).

The phenomenological method does not seek to reveal causal relationships, but rather to reveal the nature of phenomena as humanly experienced. It is a deliberate move away from quantification and testing of hypotheses. The phenomenological method, like other qualitative and quantitative methods, is a research approach encompassing five basic elements:

1. identifying the phenomenon;
2. structuring the study;
3. gathering the data;
4. analyzing the data; and
5. describing the findings.

IDENTIFYING THE PHENOMENON

A phenomenon is a circumstance that can be investigated. A phenomenon worthy of investigation in nursing science is a human circumstance related to health. The identification of a phenomenon surfaces as the nurse researcher focuses on an area of particular interest. The areas of interest in nursing science from the paradigm set forth in Chapter II of this book are in the realm of the lived experiences of structuring meaning, cocreating rhythmical patterns and cotranscending with possibles. Some phenomena for study might be: suffering, being sad, being joyful, being fearful.

STRUCTURING THE STUDY

The second element from the perspective of the phenomenological method is structuring the study plan. This includes specifying a research question that is the researcher's intent in studying a particular phenomenon, making explicit the researcher's perspective of the phenomenon, identifying a study sample and protecting the rights of subjects.

Research Question

Research questions such as "How is suffering lived for persons who are dying," "What is the meaning of being sad for persons experiencing life transitions," "What is the meaning of being fearful for persons facing surgery," or "What is being joyful like for pre-schoolers," lead the researcher to the use of the phenomenological method. These questions focus on seeking an understanding of experiences as humanly lived and reflect the meaning of health articulated in Chapter II. These questions, appropriate in light of this nursing perspective, guide the structuring of interrogative statements that encourage the subjects to share personal thoughts, perceptions, and feelings about the phenomenon in an unstructured way.

Researcher's Perspective

The researcher's beliefs about the phenomenon being studied are made explicit in the phenomenological method. Early in the planning of the study, and finally in the report of such research, the views of the researcher are made clear. The researcher describes the personal meanings of the phenomenon under study, which include beliefs from a theoretical and experiential frame of reference.

Study Sample

The study sample is drawn from a population living the experience of the phenomenon being studied. Adequacy of the sample is achieved when the researcher experiences redundancy in descriptions. Redundancy is repetition of statements regarding the phenomenon under study. For example, when a particular idea is expressed repeatedly about the same phenomenon, the researcher decides that the sample is adequate. Redundancy occurs in the descriptions of individual subjects as well as groups.

Protecting the Rights of Human Subjects

In the phenomenological method subjects are invited to respond in writing or orally, and their responses are the data of the study. The research question and the purpose of the study are discussed with the subjects who agree to participate. The nature of the study, the time commitment, and the involvement of subjects is explained, as is the option to withdraw from the study. Confidentiality and anonymity are assured. Subjects are informed that if the descriptions are published, no names will be associated with the data.

DATA GATHERING

Since the phenomenological method involves retrospective descriptions of lived experiences, the question to subjects leads them to reflect on and describe a situation or circumstance in which the experience occurred and is presently remembered.

> Describe a situation in which you experienced *suffering.* Share all the thoughts, perceptions, and feelings you can recall until you have no more to say about the situation.

An interrogatory statement such as this is given to the subjects along with an explanation, either written or oral, regarding the protection of rights. Subjects are asked to return the descriptions to the distributor or directly to the researcher. There is no specified time allotment for completing the description, and no direction to subjects other than that stated in the interrogatory invitation. The mechanics of the data gathering vary somewhat, depending on the data analysis procedure. For example, in one modification derived from the classic phenomenological method, large numbers (50–100) of anonymous descriptions are collected for analysis. In another modification smaller numbers (2–10) are collected for analysis. The subjects are known to the researcher and are invited to elaborate on the description where the researcher requires more information. Examples of both modifications are shown in Chapters IV and V of this text. After the data collection is completed, the data are initially examined and prepared for analysis.

DATA ANALYSIS

The data analysis element of the phenomenological method is rigorous, adhering strictly to a systematic approach, which compels the researcher to abide by the spirit and intent of the guiding principles of phenomenological analysis. The strict adherence is in the contemplative dwelling with the data. *Contemplative dwelling* is the undistracted reading and re-reading of the descriptions with the intent to uncover the meaning of the lived experience for the subject. The contemplative dwelling frees the researcher to be open to both the tacit and explicit messages in the data.

Essentials of the Phenomenological Method

Spiegelberg (1976) sets forth the essentials by describing the major activities that are the guiding principles of phenomenological analysis:

1. investigating the particular phenomena,
2. investigating general essences,
3. apprehending the essential relationships among essences,
4. watching modes of appearing,
5. watching the constitution of phenomena in consciousness,
6. suspending belief in the existence of the phenomena,
7. interpreting the meaning of the phenomena. (p. 659)

INVESTIGATING PARTICULAR PHENOMENA Here, three operations are included which constitute the major processes of analysis in the phenomenological method. They are *intuiting, analyzing* and *describing*. These processes are closely related and, though discrete in operation, occur simultaneously. *Intuiting* is the process of coming to know the phenomenon as described by the subject. It is a demanding activity requiring concentration and strict adherence to the surfacing meaning of the phenomenon as it shows itself in the descriptions of subjects. Each description is read in a quiet setting to minimize distractions and to allow the researcher to reflect and weigh the essences of the phenomenon as they appear. The idea of intuiting is to grasp the uniqueness of the phenomenon by openly looking, listening, and feeling. Being open to a phenomenon as it reveals itself is a difficult process for which no detailed instructions can be given. Observing persons skilled in the use of the phenomenological method as they participate in the process of intuiting is most helpful to the researcher without experience in this method (Spiegelberg, 1976).

Analyzing, the second operation in the process of investigating a phenomenon, is the strict intentional tracing of the elements and structure of the phenomenon revealed through intuiting. It explores the distinguishing characteristics of the phenomenon and its connections and relation to other phenomena. It is an attempt to uncover the constitutional elements of the phenomenon in order to come to know the whole of it, to shape its meaning as a lived experience. *Analyzing* is "the general examination of the structure of the phenomenon according to its ingredients and configuration" (Spiegelberg, 1976, p. 671).

Describing is an integral part of intuiting and analyzing. It is the process of affirming a connection between the phenomenon and everything which is denoted or connoted by way of the terms used in references to it (Spiegelberg, 1976, p. 673). Describing focuses attention on the major characteristics of the phenomenon, setting forth the essences and pointing beyond them. It is not an exhaustive process, but rather a selective one, which culminates in an elaboration of the meaning of the elements and structure of a lived experience.

The processes of intuiting, analyzing, and describing, fundamental to the phenomenological method, are processes lived all at once as the researcher dwells with subjects' descriptions of a phenomenon. These activities are not easy to accomplish and take time and persistence. Researchers who are just learning the method require supervision by one skilled in it. These fundamental processes permeate the other six activities of the method.

INVESTIGATING GENERAL ESSENCES Investigating general essences occurs by eidetic intuiting. To apprehend general essences of a phenomenon, it is necessary to examine the particulars. This is the process of interrogation of the particulars by reflecting on remembered experiences written by subjects. For example, "Using the particular red of an individual rose as a point of departure we can see it as an instance of a certain shade of red in general. But we can also see it as exemplifying redness and finally color as such" (Spiegelberg, 1976, p. 677). Thus, examining particulars leads to the apprehension of general essences.

APPREHENDING ESSENTIAL RELATIONSHIPS This process involves examining the internal relationships between the particulars within a single general essence, as well as relations among several general essences. The major goal of apprehending essential relationships is to ascertain the nature of the general essences. This is done by examining both the internal connections and connections to other essences. The process by which this is achieved is called imaginative variation (Spiegelberg, p. 680). This process has two operations; the first to omit certain components within each essence of the phenomenon completely, and the second to replace certain components with others. Both activities are directed toward answering the question: What is the nature of the essences, general and particular, of the phenomenon? If a component can be omitted without changing the nature of the essences, then it is not essential and should be omitted. If replacement components are found to be compatible with the nature of the essences of the phenomenon, they should be included in the description. Thus a deeper understanding of the phenomenon can be achieved. The phenomenon becomes more specific in fundamental meaning as the researcher engages in the operations of imaginative variation.

WATCHING MODES OF APPEARING   The systematic exploration of a phenomenon entails not only what appears, whether particular or general essences, but also the way in which things appear (Spiegelberg, 1976, p. 685). The way in which a thing appears is significant to the understanding of the phenomenon as a whole. Watching modes of appearing is an activity which focuses attention on the way a phenomenon presents itself, both to the subjects, as explicated in the descriptions and to the researcher, as the phenomenon unfolds through the *dwelling with* the subjects' descriptions. The subjects describe the general sense of the experience as well as the particular characteristics that identify the experience for them. A question like, ''How did the experience announce itself to you?'' guides the subjects to explore particular characteristics of the way in which the phenomenon presented itself to them. The researcher then dwells with these descriptions and, in the research-researcher dialectic, watches the modes of appearing as they surface from the descriptions. Each reveals a view of the phenomenon. Collectively, the descriptions reveal the various profiles of the phenomenon as it was experienced.

WATCHING THE CONSTITUTION OF PHENOMENA IN CONSCIOUSNESS   The activity of exploring how a phenomenon constitutes itself in consciousness occurs through a process of integrating the unfamiliar with the familiar. This process of constituting the phenomenon is the coming to know the general essences of the phenomenon through structuring the particulars in a way that expands the familiar. "Constitutional exploration consists of determining the way in which a phenomenon establishes itself and takes shape in our consciousness" (Spiegelberg, 1976, p. 688). To know the constitution of a phenomenon is to expand the understanding of that phenomenon. For example, the knowledge of a stranger's personality grows from the links one makes, beginning with the first impression and continuing with subsequent meetings. The connectedness among the links constitutes the pattern which is the stranger's personality (Spiegelberg, 1976, p. 689).

SUSPENDING BELIEF IN THE EXISTENCE OF THE PHENOMENA Suspending belief in existence of a phenomenon is called *bracketing*. Bracketing is the process of setting aside or detaching the meaning of the phenomenon for the researcher as opposed to the phenomenon as it appears. Bracketing is holding in abeyance the researcher's presuppositions about a phenomenon. Although the researcher makes explicit a notion of the phenomenon, and sets this notion aside when the data are approached for analysis, the researcher is aware of personal beliefs and theoretical perspectives about the phenomenon and knows that these are reflected in the analysis. It is important in "phenomenology that we consider all of the data, real or unreal or doubtful, as having equal rights, and investigate them without fear or favor" (Spiegelberg, 1976, p. 672). Bracketing, then, attempts to ensure that all available perspectives of a phenomenon are considered in uncovering the nature of the essences of that phenomenon.

INTERPRETING CONCEALED MEANINGS OF PHENOMENA Hermeneutical interpretation is the final activity in the phenomenological process. "Hermeneutics is an attempt to interpret the 'sense' of certain phenomena" (Spiegelberg, 1976, p. 695). This activity requires the researcher to dwell with the subjects' descriptions and to go beyond what is directly given" (Spiegelberg, 1976, p. 695). The researcher has discovered the given from carrying out the previous six activities of the phenomenological method. To go beyond what is given is an intuitive leap which is a shift in the level of discourse from the concrete to the abstract. The intuitive leap constitutes inferences about the concealed meanings inherent in the subjects' descriptions. This process is appropriate in that the researcher does not share in the particular experience as described, but does share in the general sense of it, as a human being. The meaning of a phenomenon is that which is sought through use of the phenomenological method, and it leads to identification of structural descriptions of that phenomenon. It is the result of intuitive seeing. These seven activities of the phenomenological method have been interpreted in several ways, two of which will be discussed here.

van Kaam Modification of the Phenomenological Method

van Kaam (1969) posited a modification for phenomenological analysis consistent with the essential activities defined by Spiegelberg (1976). These six operations of scientific explication are:

1. eliciting descriptive expressions,
2. identifying common elements,
3. eliminating those expressions not related to the phenomenon,
4. formulating a hypothetical definition of the phenomenon,
5. applying the hypothetical definition to the original descriptions,
6. identifying the structural definition.

The researcher dwells with the descriptions through the intuiting, analyzing, and describing processes, and elicits the descriptive expressions and names the common elements. A descriptive expression is a statement that completes an idea about the lived experiences. A common element is an abstract statement naming a major theme which surfaces from the descriptive expressions. To be considered a common element, a statement must be explicitly or implicitly in the majority of descriptions and compatible with all. There are usually several common elements in any phenomenological study using the van Kaam modification. The common elements are synthesized into a hypothetical definition of the phenomenon which is applied to all descriptions. Through final analysis and synthesis, a description of the phenomenon surfaces. Judges are used for verification of the descriptive expressions, common elements, and structural definitions. These judges are experienced researchers familiar with the phenomenological method. Using judges for testing and retesting the researcher's intuiting is required to provide the verification for assertions derived from phenomenological studies.

Giorgi Modification of the Phenomenological Method

Another modification of procedure for phenomenological analysis was posited by Giorgi (1970; 1979). Giorgi set forth the idea of psychology as a human science and a research method of inquiry, consistent with the idea of human science which takes into consideration Man's participation with life events. The phenomenological analysis suggested by Giorgi focuses on uncovering the meaning of lived experiences through in-depth study of subjects' descriptions. The process includes:

1. dwelling with the description,
2. returning to subject for elaboration on ambiguous areas of description,
3. identifying natural meaning unit,
4. identifying themes,
5. identifying focal meanings,
6. synthesizing of situated structural descriptions,
7. synthesizing of a general structural description.

In analyzing the data the researcher dwells with each description, identifies questions, and returns to the subject for an elaborated description. The elaborated description is studied through the processes of intuiting, analyzing, and describing. Each subject's description is examined and natural meaning units, or scenes, are identified. The scene, a unit of the description which begins and ends a thought, is examined for emerging themes, which are identified in the words of the subject and are the central elements of the scenes. Then focal meanings are identified. The focal meaning is the crystallization of the theme, which is written in the language of the researcher and shifts the level of abstraction of the theme. A synthesis of the focal meanings becomes the situated structural description of the subjects' description and thus specifies the meaning of the phenomenon from the perspective of each subject. The situated structures for all subjects are synthesized into a general structural description of the phenomenon, which is the meaning of the lived experience of the phenomenon studied from the perspective of the subjects.

DESCRIBING THE FINDINGS

Reporting a phenomenological study requires the presentation of data samples from each activity carried out by the researcher to demonstrate how the researcher moved from the subjects' descriptions to a structural definition. Because of the voluminous nature of the data, examples only are shown in a report of findings. A discussion is included with the description of findings which connects them retrospectively with the phenomenon and with the researcher's perspective, and posits non-directive propositions for research and practice. The major finding of a phenomenological study is the structural definition of the phenomenon as a lived experience.

The next two chapters present phenomenological studies which demonstrate the implementation of two different modifications of the method.

IV

The Lived Experience Of Health
A Phenomenological Study

PURPOSE

The purpose of the study presented here was to evolve a structural definition of health as it is experienced in everyday life. The rationale for choosing the phenomenological method for this study was that this method is directed toward uncovering the meaning of phenomena as humanly experienced. It is a human science method which takes into account unitary Man's participative experience with a situation and focuses on evolving structural definitions of lived experiences, such as a feeling of health.

RESEARCH QUESTION

This investigation sought to answer the question: What are the common elements in experiencing a feeling of health among several different age groups?

PHENOMENON

The phenomenon central to this study is the feeling of health. Health has been defined in a number of ways in the nursing and health-related literature by a variety of scientists and health promoters. One definition of health reveals that "health is a state of complete physical, mental, and social well-being and not merely an absence of disease or infirmity" (WHO, 1946); another states that "health is the ability of a system to respond to a wide variety of environmental challenges" (Brody and Sobel, 1979; pp. 93–94); and another says that health is a synthesis of wellness and illness (Newman, 1979); yet another says health is a state and a process of becoming an integrated whole (Roy, 1984).

RESEARCHER'S PERSPECTIVE

The researcher's perspective of a feeling of health as a lived experience is that it is an open process of becoming, experienced by Man. It is a unique experience describable only by the individual who is living it. Health is a rhythmically coconstituting process of the man-environment interrelationship. It is an intersubjective process of transcending with the possibles. The subject to subject encounters spawn different options which lead to a moving beyond. Health is not a linear entity that can be interrupted or qualified by terms such as good, bad, more, or less (Parse, 1981). It is a synthesis of values, a way of living. Health is not determined by social norms; it emerges and changes as Man structures meaning in situations (Frankl, 1967). For the researcher conducting this study, health is a lived experience, a continuously changing process in which Man knowingly participates.

SAMPLE

The sample consisted of 400 subjects, 100 between the ages of 7 and 19; 100 between 20 and 45; 100 between 46 and 65; and 100 over 66. Each group of 100 had 50 men and 50 women. These 400 subjects participated by writing descriptions of a personal situation in which a feeling of health was experienced.

PROTECTION OF SUBJECTS' RIGHTS

The subjects were informed about the nature of the study, the time commitment, and their involvement. The only demographic data requested were age and gender. No names were associated with the descriptions. Writing the description was considered consent to participate.

DATA GATHERING

The interrogatory invitation was distributed widely in colleges, universities, community agencies, and school systems and responses were returned to the researcher directly. The subjects were asked: "Describe a situation in which you experienced a feeling of health. Share your thoughts, perceptions, and feelings about the situation."

DATA ANALYSIS

The subjects' descriptions were analyzed through processes of intuiting, analyzing, and describing in the six operations of scientific explication of phenomenological analysis (van Kaam, 1969). A description of the researcher's activities follows:

1. Eliciting descriptive expressions
The researcher read and dwelled with each subject's description and, through intuiting, analyzing, and describing, decided on the descriptive expressions. The researcher then listed the expressions from each subject's descriptions. A descriptive expression is a statement that completes an idea about the lived experience.

2. Identifying common elements of experience
The researcher continued the processes of intuiting, analyzing, and describing in an effort to capture the meaning of health for the subjects by surfacing the common elements. A common element is an abstract statement describing a major theme which appears explicitly or implicitly in most descriptions and is compatible with all. All 400 subjects' descriptions were examined for general common elements; then the descriptions from each discrete age group consisting of 50 men and 50 women were examined for more specific statements of the common elements. The specific common elements arose from the general common elements and were identified in light of the descriptive expressions of each age group.

3. Eliminating those expressions not related to the phenomenon
All descriptive expressions were included for all 400 subjects.

4. Formulating a hypothetical definition of the phenomenon
Four hypothetical definitions were derived from the specific common elements and descriptive expressions of each of the four age

groups. One synthesized definition was arrived at from the general common elements of all 400 subjects' descriptions.

    5. Applying the hypothetical definition to the original descriptions

Each description was studied in relation to its specific age group's hypothetical definition and the general hypothetical definition.

    6. Identifying the structural definition

A structural definition of health for each of the four groups was identified and one structural definition from all 400 subjects' descriptions was synthesized. All of these activities were verified by two judges.

Presentation of Data

The result of the analysis from all 400 subjects is shown, and then the results from each of the four age groups. The presentation of data in the van Kaam modification involves disclosing the descriptive expressions, the common elements, and the structural definitions determined by the researcher and verified by two judges.

When the data from all 400 subjects in this study were examined, three general common elements surfaced. When these elements are described for each specific age group, they contain a greater level of specificity which is directly related to the particular descriptive expressions within the age group. The descriptive expressions are written in the language of the subject and the common elements are stated in the language of the researcher at a more abstract level of discourse.

Results—All 400 Subjects

From the descriptions of the 400 subjects, 200 men and 200 women, 762 descriptive expressions evolved. These descriptions elicited three general common elements: energy, plentitude, and harmony. An hypothetical definition was created through a synthesis of these elements. For the 400 subjects in this study, *health is harmony sparked by energy leading to plentitude.*

Results: Group 1

From the descriptions of the 100 subjects, 50 men and 50 women, under 19 years of age, 129 descriptive expressions evolved. Three specific common elements emerged from these descriptions (see Appendix A1). They are: invigorating force, constructing successfulness, and resonating clarity. The hypothetical definition was created through a synthesis of these elements. For the 100 subjects under 19 years of age in this study, *health is resonating clarity powered by an invigorating force in constructing successfulness.* An example of the descriptive expressions leading to the specific common elements follows in Table 3. For a complete list, see Appendix A1.

Results: Group 2

From the descriptions of the 100 subjects, 50 men and 50 women, between 20 and 45 years of age, 291 descriptive expressions evolved. The three specific common elements which emerged are: spirited intensity, fulfilling inventiveness, and symphonic integrity (see Appendix A2). The hypothetical definition was created through a synthesis of these elements. For the 100 subjects between 20 and 45 in this study, *health is symphonic integrity manifested in the spirited intensity of fulfilling inventiveness.* An example of the de-

TABLE 3   GROUP 1. COMMON ELEMENTS WITH DESCRIPTIVE EXPRESSIONS

INVIGORATING FORCE	CONSTRUCTING SUCCESSFULNESS	RESONATING CLARITY
1. Feels good to run and jog.	1. Feeling satisfaction at accomplishing goal	1. Feeling all is going well
2. Feeling good after strenuous exercise	2. Winning in competition with the best	2. Feeling relaxed
3. Feeling that you can do anything	3. Feeling more creative and productive	3. Sense of well-being
4. The most alive feeling I could imagine	4. Finishing a race made me glad	4. Feeling together after a swim
5. Feeling glad when riding bike up and down hills	5. Accomplishing a feat	5. Feeling happy running along with my mom
6. Enthusiastic	6. Knowing that I am producing at my highest level	6. Being with friends that value what you say
7. Running and playing	7. Ability to achieve the unexpected	7. Happy, relaxed, relieved
8. Feeling good all the time	8. Winning a competition	8. Being with others
9. Feeling totally alive and full of energy while feeling great about everything and everybody	9. Having a well-toned body	9. Free state of being
10. Running, jumping, playing football	10. Feeling of accomplishment	10. Like a spring morning—cool, breezy, sunny

scriptive expressions leading to the specific common elements follows in Table 4. For a complete list, see Appendix A2.

Results: Group 3

From the descriptions of the 100 subjects, 50 men and 50 women, between 46 and 65 years of age, 169 descriptive expressions evolved. The three specific common elements which emerged are: exhilarated potency, creating triumphs, and serene unity (see Appendix A3). The hypothetical definition was created through a synthesis of these elements. For subjects between 46 and 65 in this study, *health is serene unity lived in exhilarated potency toward creating triumphs.* An example of the descriptive expressions leading to specific common elements follows in Table 5. For a complete list, see Appendix A3.

Results: Group 4

From the descriptions of the 100 subjects, 50 men and 50 women, over 66 years of age, 173 descriptive expressions evolved. The three specific common elements which emerged are: transcendent vitality, generating completeness, and synchronous contemplation (see Appendix A4). The hypothetical definition was created through a synthesis of these elements. For the 100 subjects over 66

TABLE 4   GROUP 2. COMMON ELEMENTS WITH DESCRIPTIVE EXPRESSIONS

SPIRITED INTENSITY	FULFILLING INVENTIVENESS	SYMPHONIC INTEGRITY
1. Being enthusiastic	1. Finishing a project that takes up time	1. Being at ease
2. Catching a second wind.	2. Accomplishment	2. Feeling of worth
3. Exercising and walking	3. Winning the game of life	3. Enjoying own space at that moment
4. Feel in peak condition	4. Trying some new endeavor	4. Peaceful feeling inside while bicycling
5. Positive outlook on life	5. Feeling something enriching my life	5. A "just right" feeling about everything
6. Feeling of refreshment	6. Doing what I struggled for	6. Drinking in the beauty of the day
7. Feeling full of energy	7. Pushing a little extra	7. Peaceful attitude
8. A glowing light of energy burning brightly in my eyes	8. Feel successful as a person	8. Rhythmical, easy, warm
9. A whip the world feeling	9. Ability to extend the limits of endurance	9. Glowing and good inside
10. A surge of energy	10. Accomplishing something.	10. Feeling loved

TABLE 5   GROUP 3. COMMON ELEMENTS WITH DESCRIPTIVE EXPRESSIONS

EXHILARATED POTENCY	CREATING TRIUMPHS	SERENE UNITY
1. Laughing, singing, enjoying exercises to music	1. Satisfaction of a goal accomplished and its special memories	1. Completely at peace with myself
2. Functioning at high gear	2. Achievement of many life goals	2. Creation of the spirit of peace
3. Eager upon rising	3. Ability to do a job	3. Feeling light inside
4. Feeling great from involvement with vigorous activity	4. Having a plan for future but living one day at a time to its fullest	4. Feeling restful
5. Feeling extra good and alert	5. Pride in accomplishing planned activities	5. Being one with world
6. Walking fast	6. Ability to cope with any problems	6. Feeling of relief on hearing good news
7. Active participation in keeping fit	7. Pride and joy at accomplishing what I want to do	7. An uncluttered day
8. Had a lot of energy	8. Ability to be productive	8. A pleasant afternoon with the family
9. Felt I could lick the world	9. Feeling of accomplishment	9. General sense of everything right
10. Distinct feeling of increased alertness	10. Ability to achieve a goal	10. A certain serenity

in this study, *health is synchronous contemplation fired by transcendent vitality in generating completeness.*

An example of the descriptive expressions leading to the specific common elements follows in Table 6. For a complete list, see Appendix 6.

The hypothetical definitions, then, surfacing from the four groups are:

GROUP 1.   Health is resonating clarity powered by an invigorating force in constructing successfulness.

GROUP 2.   Health is symphonic integrity manifested in the spirited intensity of fulfilling inventiveness.

GROUP 3.   Health is serene unity lived in exhilarated potency toward creating triumphs.

GROUP 4.   Health is synchronous contemplation fired by transcendent vitality in generating completeness.

These hypothetical definitions were found compatible with the subjects' descriptions in the respective age groups and were therefore accepted as the structural definitions of health for each age group. The hypothetical definition of health for the 400 subjects that is compatible with all 400 descriptions is: *Health is harmony sparked*

TABLE 6   GROUP 4. COMMON ELEMENTS WITH DESCRIPTIVE EXPRESSIONS

TRANSCENDENT VITALITY	GENERATING COMPLETENESS	SYNCHRONOUS CONTEMPLATION
1. Grateful for vitality	1. Able to accomplish extensive household tasks	1. Blessed with good health
2. Vibrant and full of zip	2. Immense satisfaction	2. Real peace of mind brought about by making decisions and sticking to them
3. Feeling of aliveness	3. Completing all plans on time	3. Awareness of time fades away
4. Excellent feeling	4. No task is too difficult	4. Feeling of thankfulness to God
5. Feeling euphoric on a bright clear day	5. Participating in productive activity	5. People loving and caring for me
6. Great, wonderful feeling	6. Full days work; no disabilities	6. Freedom from worry
7. Being able to sleep and wake up refreshed	7. Can do regular work	7. Being all right
8. Exercise everyday	8. Drive by myself	8. Walking, looking, listening to the words—sounds that remind me of another lifetime
9. Keeping active	9. Being able to perform my duties	9. When I go to see my son and granddaughter
10. Steps are light without troubles—when I feel well—those are my tall days	10. Being able to participate and achieve my goals	10. Remain active in social life with husband

by energy leading to plentitude. This was accepted as the structural definition of health for the 400 subjects in this study.

DISCUSSION OF FINDINGS

The purpose of this study was to evolve a structural definition of the lived experience of health using van Kaam's phenomenological modification. For the 400 subjects in this study, the lived experience of health is harmony sparked by energy leading to plentitude. This is the structural definition of health which surfaced from this study. Other structural definitions of health, which reflect the general common elements of harmony, energy, and plentitude and show the greater specificity of each of the four age groups, emerged from the analyses as indicated above.

Harmony-Energy-Plentitude

Harmony was revealed slightly differently for each group in the descriptions that led to the common elements. In group 1, resonating clarity was revealed in the nature of the expressions which showed a clear rhythmical process. In group 2, symphonic integrity was revealed in the sense of being in tune with the world. From group 3, serene unity surfaced from the descriptive statements related to restfulness. For group 4, synchronous contemplation was revealed as reflective rhythmical statements were made.

Energy was revealed differently in the descriptions of all four groups. In group 1, invigorating force was evident in the explicit expressions which were consistently related to movement and sports. Spirited intensity, the specific common element for group 2, surfaced from statements that showed a kind of growing intensity with life. For group 3, exhilarated potency articulated the meaning which generally focused on being active and highly alert. Transcendant vitality, in group 4, surfaced from statements that related to moving beyond the actual, looking back, and looking forward.

Plentitude surfaced in increasingly diverse ways in the descriptive expressions leading to the common elements in the four age groups. In group 1, it was revealed as constructing successfulness in the comments related to setting up goals and working hard toward accomplishments. Fulfilling inventiveness, from group 2, reflects the focus on accomplishing something through struggle. Creating triumphs, from group 3, arose from consistent statements related to pride in achievement. For group 4, generating completeness was revealed in expressions which focused on being productive.

Man-Living-Health

The structural definitions identified in this study correspond to the principles of Man-Living-Health (Parse, 1981). The themes of rhythmicity, transcendence, and meaning are reflected in the common elements of the definitions of health evolving from this study.

Harmony, specified in resonating clarity, symphonic integrity, serene unity, and synchronous contemplation, is the element clearly linked to the theme of rhythmicity and the second principle of Man-Living-Health (Parse, 1981). This principle states: "Cocreating rhythmical patterns of relating is living the paradoxical unity of revealing-concealing and enabling-limiting while connecting separating" (Parse, 1981, p. 50). The elements specified reflect the rhythmical connecting-separating in the Man-environment interchange.

Being in tune with the world is implied by ideas such as resonating, symphonic, serene, and synchronous. These all relate to rhythmical patterns that have an ebb and flow, a calmly changing movement which encompasses both the sameness and the difference in change. The movement rings with clarity and wistful contemplation in serene unity. There is a peaceful, restful feeling of oneness in harmony. Harmony described thus is an element of the lived experience of health.

Energy, specified in invigorating force, spirited intensity, exhilarated potency, and transcendent vitality, is linked to the theme of transcendence and the third principle of Man-Living-Health (Parse, 1981). The principle states: "Cotranscending with the possibles is powering unique ways of originating in the process of transforming" (Parse, 1981, p. 55). The elements specified reflect a powering, a pushing-resisting, and a moving beyond. This powering happens through an intensity that is a potent, vital force of life. It is enlivening and points to a transforming to what is not yet. There is a vigor and thrust implied in the elements that relate to powering as essential for transcending. Transcending is moving beyond the actual through powering by jogging, running, and laughing, as unique ways of originating in the process of transforming. Energy identified thus is an element of health as a lived experience.

Plentitude, specified in constructing successfulness, fulfilling inventiveness, creating triumphs, and generating completeness, is connected to the theme of meaning and the first principle of Man-Living-Health (Parse, 1981). The principle states: "Structuring meaning multidimensionally is cocreating reality through the languaging of valuing and imaging" (Parse, 1981, p. 42). The elements specified reflect the languaging of valuing through successes, inventions, triumphs, and completion of plans. Meaning is given to valued projects as they are imaged and languaged through efforts to reach goals. Man structures meaning through choosing reality from multidimensional experiences and these choices are lived in constructing, fulfilling, creating, and generating what is not yet. Man images valued possibles and languages these possibles in concrete expressions leading to a sense of plentitude. Plentitude refers to the meaning given to life projects, winnings, and accomplishments. It reflects the languaging of valued dreams through successful achievements. Plentitude defined thus is an element of the lived experience of health.

Results of the study can be generalized only to the subjects participating in this study. It can be noted, however, that the structural definitions of health are clearly different from those found in most nursing and health-related literature. The researcher's perspective was set forth early in the study and, though bracketed for the analysis, was reflected in the analysis as expected in the inevitable research-researcher engagement. The definitions of health arising from this study are compatible with the researcher's perspective in that they reveal health as a process of becoming, experienced by each individual in a way that is not linked to social expectations. They reflect the Man-environment energy interchange which is cocreated in rhythmical harmony toward transcendence. The definitions evolved from this study are consistent with the meaning of health articulated in the theory of Man-Living-Health (Parse, 1981) and they support the notion that health is not experienced as a linear entity but rather is a value one lives. The elements present in the structural definitions of health are coherent with the theory of Man-Living-Health. The structural definitions of health arising from this study, as demonstrated through discussion of the elements, correspond to the principles of Man-Living-Health, thus providing evidence of support for the theory.

V

THE LIVED EXPERIENCE OF
PERSISTING IN CHANGE
A PHENOMENOLOGICAL STUDY*

PURPOSE

This study was designed to generate a structural description of the phenomenon, *persisting in change even though it is difficult*. The structural description will be synthesized from essences of the phenomenon. *Persisting in change even though it is difficult* is a lived experience of health. This phenomenon was of interest to the researcher in view of a personal work-related situation. The methodology was chosen in that it is directed toward uncovering the meaning of a phenomenon as humanly lived.

RESEARCH QUESTION

This investigation sought to answer the question: What is the structural description of the lived experience of *persisting in change even though it is difficult*.

PHENOMENON

Persisting in change even though it is difficult, the phenomenon of this study, is a way of being with a situation. With any situation

---

*Extrapolated from a research study completed by Lisabeth K. Kraynie and reported here with permission.

one may choose to persist in spite of the difficulty inherent in the living out of that choice. *Persisting even though it is difficult* is one pattern of relating which may be chosen from myriad possibilities. It is lived as one participates with the world through personal valuing. Thus, persisting in a difficult situation is a lived experience of health.

RESEARCHER'S PERSPECTIVE

From the researcher's perspective, *persisting even though it is difficult* is a way of powering the enabling-limiting of valuing. Powering is lived in relation to one's view of a situation and to one's values, beliefs, or goals in a situation. Tillich (1954) writes of the phenomenology of power, "Power is real only in its actualization, in the encounter of other bearers of power and in the ever-changing balance which is the result of these encounters. . . . Everybody and everything has changes and must take risks, because his and its power of being remains hidden if actual encounters do not reveal it" (p. 41).

Parse (1981) describes powering as a pattern of pushing-resisting lived in the struggle and tension of every encounter. In each situation a change in the pushing-resisting tension and emerging conflict presents possibilities and opportunities for new choices and "for affirming being in spite of non-being" (pp. 57-79). Raths, et al., (1978) describes valuing as "choosing, prizing, and acting" on those choices (p. 28). Parse (1981) states that "since one cannot be all things at once, in choosing one is both enabled and limited" (p. 53). As an individual chooses to persist in difficulty, that individual is affirming belief in the values inherent in that situation and in the values of staying with that situation in spite of difficulty.

van Kaam (1972) relates the staying with one's chosen values to persistent willingness as one lives originality. He writes, ". . . it is not enough to know what road I should take among the many possible roads offered to me, I must walk that road and keep walking" (pp. 4-5). For this researcher, persisting in a difficult situation is lived, then, in relation to man's unique valuing of staying-with as choices are made which enable and limit all at once.

The researcher's experience of *persisting in change even though it is difficult* follows:

> Over the past five years I had developed a fine home health agency which was the larger component of a two-section hospital department. I had invested much energy in my work and felt that my agency was a

reflection of myself. I am proud of it and of those who work with and for me. We maintain high standards and as a result the agency is well thought of by patients, families, hospital personnel, administrators, the medical staff, and the community.

During the past year and a half, the performance of the personnel of a second component of our hospital department began to deteriorate in direct relationship to the attitude of and the pending retirement of the department chief. Because of our close intra-departmental relationship, most hospital personnel were not aware of the departmental divisions and therefore they attributed this poor performance to my agency. I began to be approached for a solution of the problems thus created by the others. As I was not responsible for those people and their chief denied that any problem existed, and, in fact, encouraged and participated in the problematic behavior, I became very frustrated with the situation. I felt helpless in that there was no way to solve the problems short of retirement of the chief. I was angry that my people were being blamed for things with which they had nothing to do. While I knew that eventually I would be responsible for both components and would be able to bring the whole department to our agency standard level, there was no way of knowing when that would happen. The department chief was already three years beyond the retirement age which had been in effect before the change by the Government to seventy years. The longer this went on, the more difficult the situation became. The chief became more and more difficult and unkind to me as time went on and was running out for her. We had had a good working relationship and I genuinely liked her as a person. In view of our long previous relationship, I was very hurt by her actions. I had no way of knowing if she would stay two more years. And, if she did, I didn't know if I wanted to continue living in this extremely difficult situation. I was torn between wanting out of the day-to-day stress and wanting to stay and preserve my previous work and also to accept the challenge of making the whole department good. At times I wanted to leave and yet I didn't know if another job would be the same or better. Administration wanted me to stay and finally decided to present to her three options: Staying on as a staff member, staying one month and finishing the year as a consultant, or leaving immediately. In the final period of this time of difficulty, I felt very sad and depressed—powerless. My heart was heavy and yet I knew that I did want to be able to work out the solutions to the departmental problems. It was not easy. As administration decided on the final approach, they also decided that I should present the options in order to make clear that I would require the former chief's support if she chose to stay as staff member and that I would be in charge. This seemed an unbelievable hurdle that I must cross with the end finally in sight if she left and the possibility of an even more difficult situation if she stayed. I knew inside that I must continue and did in fact persist and carried out the plan. The former chief threatened the hospital with an age discrimination suit, but did leave. I felt an overwhelming relief and also sadness at the end of this time. I was not happy then, but encouraged that now I could begin to repair the damage of that difficult time. I am now, several months later, beginning to feel good about the department and the subsequent work I have done to bring it to where it should be.

SAMPLE

Two subjects were invited to participate in the study. Both were professional women between the ages of twenty-five and thirty. Each was educated at the master's level. Both were known to the researcher and were asked to participate because of the researcher's knowledge of their ability to express their ideas. The sample size was limited to two descriptions.

PROTECTION OF SUBJECTS' RIGHTS

The subjects were asked to:

Write a description of a situation in which you experienced sticking with something even though it was difficult.

The subjects were given a short verbal description of the phenomenological method of research. They were invited to answer the question and to include all of their thoughts, feelings, and perceptions related to the experience. No attempt was made to influence the type of situation they described, so that the description would clearly be the subject's perspective of the phenomenon. The issues of informed consent, withdrawal, and confidentiality were addressed and their written descriptions served as consent to participate. It was also explained to the subjects that after their descriptions had been read they would be asked to elaborate certain portions of them. They were informed that no names would be used in association with the data.

DATA GATHERING

The question was given to each of the subjects and the descriptions were returned directly to the researcher. The researcher then read each description several times in order to sense the meaning of the whole and to identify the areas for elaboration. Each subject was then asked to elaborate certain areas of the descriptions. These elaborations were inserted into the original descriptions, and appear in parentheses in the raw data. This completed the data collection process.

DATA ANALYSIS

Analysis of the data was begun using the Giorgi (1975) modification. This method incorporates the rigorous process of intuiting—of dwelling with the data, analyzing, and describing the unfolding of the meaning while staying true to the things themselves in an all-at-once process of emerging meaning. The following process was adhered to:

1. identification of the natural meaning units,
2. identification of themes,
3. identification of focal meanings,
4. synthesis of situated structural descriptions,
5. synthesis of a general structural description.

The subjects' elaborated descriptions were divided into naturally occurring meaning units, or scenes. The theme that is inherent in each scene was described in the language of the subject. As the researcher dwelled with each theme, new meanings surfaced to create the focal meanings. The transition from themes to focal meanings represents a shift in level of discourse to the abstract. For each description, focal meanings were synthesized into a situated structural description which reflected the meaning of the phenomenon from the perspective of the subject, but in the language of the researcher. The two situated structural descriptions were synthesized into a general structural description which is the meaning of the phenomenon as it emerged from the lived experience of both subjects.

Each of the subjects chose a major life event to describe the experience of persisting in difficulty. One chose to describe her divorce from her first husband, including the year preceding the divorce. The other subject described her difficulty in convincing her parents to allow her to leave home for college to obtain a bachelor's degree in nursing.

The elaborated descriptions, the themes, the focal meanings, situated structures, and the synthesized general description follow.

Subject #1

Elaborated Description #1

Persistence and final decision making has never come easy for me. However, during one period in my life it became essential that I develop and utilize these qualities to their utmost. This period encompassed the year preceding my divorce from my first husband.

Theme #1

Persistence and final decision making were not easy for the subject. During the year preceding her divorce it was essential for the subject to develop and utilize these qualities to their utmost.

Focal Meaning

For this subject the experience of persisting occurred when she divorced her first husband.

Elaborated Description #2

We met at college during our sophomore year. We both majored in the same field. Throughout college we were very competitive. (I guess, I'd always gotten better grades than my husband and I was a more competitive person to begin with than he and it was just hard—being in the same field—I'm sure we would have been competitive regardless. My second husband and I are competitive. Competitiveness with my first husband was at times frustrating. It was a frustrating feeling—it made me anxious, it caused me to feel anxious a lot of the time—being competitive with someone I had such a close relationship with. However, since I came out lower on such a few occasions it didn't cause me to be overwhelmingly frustrated).†

Theme #2

Having met during their sophomore year and majored in the same field, the subject and her future husband were very competitive throughout college. The subject was the more competitive person who was frustrated and anxious because of the competitiveness with someone with whom she was so close. The frustration was not overwhelming since the subject seldom came out lower.

Focal Meaning

In the closeness of the husband-wife relationship, the subject struggled to prove herself better but was unchallenged in the process.

Elaborated Description #3

I went for my M.A. degree, and my husband went to work as a speech therapist upon graduation. Even though we were separated for that

---

†Parenthetical inclusion indicates elaboration.

year, I dated no one else. My husband and I remained best friends and in love. We became engaged and were married at the completion of my graduate work. Because it was difficult for my husband to find a job with a B.S. degree, he kept his job and I took a position with him in the public schools. In many ways I resented that because I had just spent much time and effort in being trained for hospital work which I loved.

Theme #3

The subject and future husband were separated while she went for her M.A. degree and he worked as a speech therapist for a year. They remained in love and were married at the completion of the subject's graduate work. The subject took a position in the schools because her husband had difficulty finding a job with only a B.S. degree. The subject resented this because of the time and energy spent learning hospital work which she loved.

Focal Meaning

The subject experienced resentment at being imposed upon to give up a prized activity for the good of the husband.

Elaborated Description #4

However, despite this my husband and I were very compatible and day-to-day living on an "at times" superficial basis went extremely well. We always found humor in things. Looking back on it we spent most of our time laughing and being very happy. He did everything within his power to please me.

Theme #4

The subject and her husband were compatible and living well on a superficial basis. They were happy and her husband did everything in his power to please the subject.

Focal Meaning

The subject experienced a sense of superficial lightness and compatibility in the day-to-day living with the other.

Elaborated Description #5

I was not accustomed to doing housework but by nature my husband was a perfectionist regarding housework and decorating but not so professionally motivated as me. This disturbed me for he was content for me to make more money than him and he in return assumed all household duties. (I was real comfortable with it. I had never done household things—even at college my roommate just did things instead of teaching me how to do it and so I moved from my grandmother doing my laundry and things to my roommate and then to my husband. Really it didn't bother me. He would say, ''These baseboards need done'' and it hadn't even occurred to me that we had baseboards. That almost satisfied me because I didn't have the desire to get into it.)

Theme #5

The subject was not accustomed to housework while her husband was a perfectionist in housework and decorating and assumed all household duties. Her husband was not professionally motivated and was content for the subject to make more money which disturbed her. The subject had no desire to do housework as others had always done it for her. The subject was real comfortable and almost satisfied with her husband doing housework.

Focal Meaning

The subject experienced ambivalence at being knotted together with her husband in a complementary way.

Elaborated Description #6

Appearance-wise, my husband was almost immaculate. He always encouraged me to buy clothes or go to a hair stylist. He always put me on a pedestal. I was the first and only girl he had dated seriously. I also admired him. He was much different from previous boyfriends—a football player and a radical. He was kind, gentle, giving, loving, and very domestic. Since I am an only child I felt that one reason why my family loved him so was because he thought the world of me and just stepped in and took their place in caring for me. Being cared for came easy to me. His family was extremely warm and also loving. His two brothers provided me with attention and a relationship I never had since I was an only child. His father and I were particularly close since his only daughter died many years earlier. In short, we had a very convenient and amicable marriage where much love was shared between us and our families.

Theme #6

The subject's husband was immaculate and encouraged her to buy clothes and go to a hair stylist. The subject was placed on a pedestal by her husband and admired him in return. Subject's family loved her husband because he cared for her. Being cared for came easily for the subject. Her husband's family was warm and loving. The marriage was convenient and amicable with much love shared between the subject and husband and their families.

Focal Meaning

Before the marriage the subject viewed self as entering into an ideal marital situation.

Elaborated Description #7

One year after our marriage I became restless in the schools and encouraged my husband to pursue his master's degree. He was uncertain of what he wanted to do with his life which upset me. He did not feel that he wanted to pursue an M.A. in speech since he did not want to compete with my past record or with me professionally in the future. Therefore, it was I who finally suggested that he obtain his M.Ed. in deaf education. The fact that I had to decide for him angered me but we never openly fought about it. He was accepted and therefore we moved. I luckily found a clinical position which I was pleased with and which supported us during his time at school. While in school he frequently sought my help and lacked confidence in his performance despite receiving excellent grades. His lack of confidence was very frustrating to me for I wanted him to graduate and do well professionally.

Theme #7

The subject became restless in the schools and encouraged her husband to pursue his master's degree. The husband did not want to compete with the subject. The subject suggested he obtain his M.Ed. in deaf education. The subject was angered by having to decide for him but did not fight about it. The subject worked in a clinical position and supported them. Her husband frequently sought her help as he lacked confidence despite excellent grades. The subject was frustrated by his lack of confidence as she wanted him to do well professionally.

Focal Meaning

Even when the husband responds to the subject's direction, the subject is disappointed in her husband as he falls short of her expectations.

Elaborated Description #8

In addition to my husband's lack of self confidence and lack of professional drive, he was never very physically affectionate. Initially, we had experienced sexual difficulties which I hoped would improve with time. However, these problems persisted. These difficulties, however, always seemed to balance themselves by his kindness and warmth. He was romantic in the sense that he frequently gave me flowers, cards, remembered dates I had forgotten, and showered me with gifts. I remember critizing him for being too materialistic. By the third year of our marriage, I had begun convincing myself that this was all there was to marriage—sex and love. Being married to him was very convenient and very comfortable. He was very easy to love because he gave his love so freely.

Theme #8

The subject and her husband had sexual difficulties which the subject hoped would improve with time. The husband was not physically affectionate though this was balanced for the subject by his showing kindness and warmth through flowers, cards, and gifts. The subject criticized this as materialistic and saw marriage as only sex and love. The subject saw the marriage as convenient and comfortable since the husband was easy to love and gave love freely.

Focal Meaning

Even though the husband expresses outward signs of affection, the subject was disappointed because he did not meet her expectations.

Elaborated Description #9

My husband was always a very very private person and had no close, close friends. We shared friends and were best friends. We shared all social activities and participated in everything as a couple.

Theme #9

The subject's husband was a private person with no close friends. The couple shared friends and all social activities and were best friends.

Focal Meaning

The subject experienced self as bound in a paired relationship.

Elaborated Description #10

Toward the end of the M.Ed. program, tensions began to mount. All of the above described feelings and frustrations of my life with him began to become magnified. (I think my feelings of frustration—oh—I just wanted him to take hold of his life and he was just very willing to let me do the moving—as far as what he was going to be and where we were going to be and I just wanted him to take hold of some of that. I felt like I had the most responsibility, number one, to make him something professionally and maintaining our marriage. He was very complacent and he was just very happy with the way things were. It was frustrating, I felt very tense a lot of times. I was so overwhelmed at times because I wanted to have children. I wanted to take the lesser responsibility for breadwinning and things like that. For him, children did not, were not one of his goals. I saw no end in sight.)

Theme #10

Tensions mounted as subject's feelings and frustrations were magnified. The subject wanted her husband to take hold of his life. The subject had most responsibility for her husband's profession and their marriage. The subject was tense and wanted children and less responsibility for breadwinning. The subject's husband was complacent and happy the way things were. The subject saw no end in sight.

Focal Meaning

The subject experienced being on a perpetual treadmill of increasing responsibility which magnified the growing conflict in the husband-wife relationship.

Elaborated Description #11

Looking back, this was probably due to my increased self-assertiveness and less of a need to be cared for. I was assuming increased responsibility at work and at home for family members who were ill. I began to feel for the first time in my life a sense of independence. (It felt good. I was real surprised at myself for having developed it. I had led a sheltered life and for the first time it felt like I was responsible for myself. And I could be responsible for myself—for the first time I was looking out for other people. In a sense, I had always cared and loved them, but I was assuming responsibility. At work I became the coordinator of the program and I enjoyed that feeling of responsibility. I enjoyed having my grandmother ask my opinion.)

Theme #11

The subject was increasingly self-assertive and had less need to be cared for. The subject assumed more responsibility at work and with ill family members and had a good feeling of independence. The subject was surprised and enjoyed the feeling of responsibility.

Focal Meaning

The subject experienced joy with competence and power in taking on new responsibilities.

Elaborated Description #12

We began to argue over small things, which we never did. Realistically, I instigated most arguments as a way of venting my frustration and anger over the important issues without going into them. My husband never wanted to talk seriously about our sexual or other marital problems. He felt they only existed in my mind. (I just felt very angry. He would infuriate me. He always said everything was fine. Of course, everything was fine on a superficial surface level. We cared very much for each other but he just wasn't looking at the things I confronted him with. One, the assuming of more responsibility, wanting more affection, wanting to improve my sexual relations, and he just thought, "Oh, it's all fine" and he just kind of brushed over it and I would just get so angry, so, so angry—I guess just angry.)

Theme #12

The subject instigated arguments over small things as a way of venting frustration and anger over the issues of sexual or other marital problems. The subject was infuriated because her husband would not talk, saying the problems existed in the subject's mind and everything was fine. Though superficially everything was fine and they cared for each other, the husband would not look at the subject's desire for more affection and improved sexual relations.

Focal Meaning

The subject experienced suffocating helplessness at not being heard by her husband.

Elaborated Description #13

Tensions continued to build and we separated for one month. I began to see a counselor but my husband refused. We missed each other dearly and went back together only to separate again after two months for a two month period. Each separation was my idea. I had to be persistent that I needed time. This killed me because I never had lived alone and I was physically and emotionally afraid. I also missed my husband who was my best friend. (It was so hard. In a lot of ways I didn't really want the separation because I leaned on him. I was just trying to make myself forget and I would say, "Oh, everyone has problems, you're never going to find a perfect marriage and this is the best that you can do. He is a good person." So all of those things balanced with all of my frustrations and other feelings struck a pretty even balance and therefore I think if it had been heavier one way or the other, I don't think I would have had to feel that I had to be so persistent internally because I would have just rationally said, "Oh, look this marriage isn't good," and would have ended it years before. The fact that it was so even—I really had to persist in myself and do it. And because I had never lived alone and I was afraid of losing him. Not only his physical presence—I was afraid of somebody breaking in or doing something. I was alone and it would have been very easy at that time to just go back to him and forget our differences. I persisted in the separation, but then, I did go back thinking, you know—it was crazy because the more I was away from him the more I missed him. He was my best friend as well as my husband. I just missed him when I was away from him. The feelings of just missing him tended to override my feelings of why I had left him but then I would be with him no more than a day and they would all come back and I would realize I had to be truthful with myself. It just wasn't going to work out. Because we'd fall back into the same patterns and I'd be frustrated again. It was really difficult to make that decision. And the other times it was hard too, going back and forth, back and forth. Since he was ignoring that there were problems, it made my persistence even greater. He was admitting to nothing. I had to really struggle and persist that we did have problems to even make him realize what I was talking about. Finally I realized that the marriage was not working nor would it ever work. I knew I had to end it. My husband never would. (I think after our separations, the final time that we separated, I thought and said to myself, "This is it—the final time." And then in a week or so I really missed him and I really had to convince myself that "Yes, I do miss him but I cannot continue to put him and myself through this because I know that as soon as I go back—the situation hasn't changed and I know that I'm going to put myself and him through this separation business again.") Despite my persistence for him to be realistic and talk to me about our future, he continued to send flowers and plead with me not to file for a divorce. Although I realized that I must be strong and follow my best instincts, I was pulled to him, a person I still loved very much as well as his family who wanted us to stay together. My family was supportive of me, but continued to voice their deep feelings for him. Although I had primarily carried the financial load, I looked to him for security, happiness and love, but now to do what I felt was right I had to sacrifice everything and break up the physical comfort afforded by our home together.

Theme #13

The subject and her husband separated two times and missed each other. The separations were the subject's idea as she needed time. The subject had never been alone and was physically and emotionally afraid. The subject leaned on her husband and in a lot of ways didn't want the separation. The subject sometimes felt the marriage was the best she could do and that this struck a pretty even balance with her frustrations. The subject felt that if the balance had been heavier one way or the other she would not have had to be so internally persistent. The subject went back and forth between missing him and her feelings of why she had left him. The subject knew that the marriage would not work and she had to end it, that her husband never would. The subject knew she must be strong in spite of her husband and their families and that she must sacrifice security, happiness, and love to do what she felt was right.

Focal Meaning

The subject was torn between wanting to be separated and wanting to be married.

Elaborated Description #14

Of course, to all of our friends and family who did not know of the private circumstances of our difficulties, I was the villain who wanted to destroy his life. I lost all of our mutual friends as a result. (That's probably one of the hardest things that made persisting so difficult because I'd never been the villain. I'd always done the right things, had a nice relationship with my friends, my family, and at school. I'd always been the good guy and really had never done anything to make anybody unhappy and now all of a sudden all of my friends and my family were questioning. How could I do this to him and to us? Being the villain just hurt me. My family understood, but his did not. It was just a very hurtful time. It was a totally different situation than I'd ever been in in my life.) But inside I knew that through two separations, marriage would never be quite right for us again. Therefore, I filed for a dissolution of our marriage.

Theme #14

The subject was the villain who wanted to destroy her husband's life to their friends and families and lost all of their friends. The subject had never been the villain—always the good guy—so this was the hardest thing and made persisting so difficult. This was a different, hurtful situation with everyone questioning how the subject could do this. But the subject knew the marriage would never be right and filed for dissolution.

Focal Meaning

The subject experienced turmoil with the clash of perspectives which emerged in choosing divorce.

Elaborated Description #15

Countless times I wavered and called the attorney with thoughts of reconsidering, but in the final analysis my heart told me that I must go through with it. My brain, on the other hand, said that I was crazy for giving up such a wonderful man whom I loved in many ways, my friends, and his much loved family. (We had separate apartments and he would come and knock on my door and say he didn't come to discuss but brought flowers and he came when I had become ill. Just to see him and be with him when he didn't come to yell, but came to help me just made me waver—made me remember all the good times we had had and what all I was giving up—just what a good person he was. He would say, "Just tell me you don't love me and I'll be able to accept this." I just couldn't give him that satisfaction because I did still love him and I do still love him. It was driving me crazy—to see him and remembering all of our good times together made me waver. If he were a son of a gun or a bad husband, I don't think I would have wavered. His only crime, our only problem was that he wasn't everything that I felt that I needed. I married him knowing that he, or we, had these faults together and expected them to get better but when things didn't, that's when things got shaky. But once again the wavering came in so much because he was such a good man to give up. I guess a lot of times I would feel like I was drowning—almost dying, a part of me was dying because he just meant so much to me. And I would feel like I was trying to save our marriage—oh, no, I can't say that, at the end I wasn't trying to save our marriage. I would feel like—if he and I are divorced, then, how is my life going to be? I just couldn't imagine life without him and yet I couldn't imagine going through the rest of my life with him. I just felt real unsure of myself in all kinds of ways. I felt I was ugly, just— unprofessional, I felt my whole life was going down the tubes. Then I would waver and have periods when I wouldn't be unsure. I would know this is what I should do. It was an unsure feeling, scary, for sure.)

Theme #15

The subject wavered countless times. Her heart told her to go through with it while her brain said she was crazy for giving up a wonderful man whom she still loved in many ways, his friends, and his family. The subject remembered the good times, what she was giving up and what a good person her husband was. The subject could not give her husband the satisfaction of saying she didn't love him. The subject felt her husband's only problem was not being everything she needed. The subject had married knowing this and expected the faults to get better. The subject felt she was drowning—almost dying. The subject could not imagine life without her husband or going through the rest of her life with him. The subject felt unsure, ugly, unprofessional, and as if her whole life was going down the tubes. At other times the subject was not unsure and knew the divorce was what she should do.

Focal Meaning

The subject experienced self as whirlpooled into hopelessness as reflected in her own inadequacies in her relationship with another.

Elaborated Description #16

In the months preceding the actual divorce, my husband plagued me with guilt for ruining his life, violating his trust, and hurting his family. He threatened to end his life which surprisingly angered me for it was an extension of his need for me to give his life direction when I so needed him to assume more responsibility for himself as well as me professionally and emotionally.

Theme #16

The subject's husband plagued her with guilt for ruining his life, violating his trust, and hurting his family. The subject was angry when he threatened to end his life when she needed him to be responsible for them.

Focal Meaning

The subject experienced disdain for her husband when he continued to fall short of her expectations.

Elaborated Description #17

On the day of our divorce, I was a shambles. I no longer felt that I knew what I wanted. I cried through the divorce proceedings. When the judge asked if I was sure if I wanted the marriage dissolved, I couldn't answer but the attorney replied for me. (I was just emotionally and physically a wreck. I just felt a mess and emotionally a shambles. I was feeling this tremendous guilt. I was feeling afraid that this was it. I had done this all by myself, my husband didn't want it. I thought, why couldn't he want it too because if he wanted it too it would be less hard for me. He never wanted it, not for a minute and it was like pulling teeth to get him to sign the papers. I was alone and just physically and mentally down.)

Theme #17

The subject was a shambles on the day of the divorce. The subject was emotionally and physically a wreck, crying and unable to answer the judge. The subject felt guilty and alone because she had done this and her husband had never wanted it. The subject questioned why. It would have been less hard if he had wanted it, too.

Focal Meaning

When faced with the realization of the finality of terminating the relationship, the subject was overwhelmed with the consequences of her choice.

Elaborated Description #18

Surprisingly, my husband was very kind and strong. The judge stated that he would hold the papers till Monday before processing and stated that if we changed our minds to give him a call and he would destroy them. We left the building together. When we reached the door he said, "Let's tear up the papers, let's start over." Despite my sense of isolation and sadness and love for him at that moment I persisted in my decision to proceed with the divorce. I feel that I have never had to acquire such strength in making a decision and "sticking to it" as on that day. (I must admit, when it was done, immediately—that minute—I didn't feel relieved, not right after it was done. It was still—I could have killed the judge because he was just real unsure whether I really wanted this and I was just overcome. It was funny that on that day it was my husband who was the strong one. He really helped me. I was still wavering even after it was done. My husband was saying to start over and by that time I had gotten hold of myself and said, "No, I don't think we can do that." It wasn't until I flew to Chicago on Sunday and he and I were not in the same town that I began to feel good about it. I felt that I finally had made it. Once I got away from the drama of the courtroom and the emotional feelings I had about him I was able to put the whole thing in perspective. I realized my reasons for persisting. Later that week I actually felt good about having done it. I felt—well—it's done, and I lived through it and I did it on my own in spite of him and his family and his friends. I still did what I thought was best—best for me and for him. For the first time in a year and a half I felt like I didn't have a dark cloud over me. I didn't have to wake up in the night and think— am I going to have to go through with this again? It was like my decision was done and I think that this feeling was intensified because I had so much wavering. It wasn't until it was actually done and filed that I felt good about persisting. It was a very good feeling. I still had bad times, but—. It was satisfying. I was satisfied that I had done the right thing. I felt less guilt, too, because I was able to look at it more realistically. I had persisted through it and I realized that it just wasn't all my fault. Feeling relieved, less guilty, and also just feeling contentment with myself—that I had done something all by myself in spite of all the frustrating things from my husband—pressure.)

Theme #18

The subject was surprised that her husband was strong and kind to her. When her husband wanted to start over, the subject persisted in her decision to proceed with the divorce even though she felt isolated and sad. This took great strength and "sticking to it." The subject still wavered after it was done. It was not until they were in separate towns that the subject felt good about it—that she had finally made it. She was able to put the divorce in perspective. The subject had an intense feeling of doneness, satisfaction that she had done the right thing, relief, less guilt, and a feeling of contentment with herself. After a year and a half, there was not a dark cloud over her.

Focal Meaning

The subject experienced relief and satisfaction as the overwhelming experience of uncertainty and aloneness was tempered with time.

The focal meanings were synthesized into a situated structural description for subject number 1, as follows:

Situated Structural Description #1

The subject in this situation viewed herself as entering into the ideal marital situation. *Persisting even though it is difficult* occurred when she divorced her first husband. In the closeness of their relationship, she was very competitive and struggled to prove herself better. She was unchallenged in this process. Day-to-day living was experienced as having a superficial lightness and compatibility. Her husband assumed the household duties while she made more money professionally. She experienced ambivalence at being knotted together with her husband in this complementary way.

Because her husband was limited in job choice, she took a position in the schools after earning her masters degree for hospital work. She resented being imposed upon to give up this prized activity for the good of her husband. Even though he responded to her direction and obtained his masters degree and also expressed outward affection, she was disappointed because he didn't meet her expectations. They shared all friends and activities and she felt bound in a paired relationship.

She felt increasing responsibility which seemed as if she was on a perpetual treadmill—which magnified the conflict in their relationship. As she took on new responsibilities she began to experience joy in an emerging sense of competence and power.

Her husband would not acknowledge the conflict as she experienced suffocating helplessness since he would not hear her. She was torn between wanting separation and wanting marriage. She saw herself as trapped on a treadmill, helpless, and alone. She experienced turmoil with the clash of perspectives—husband, wife, and family and friends—as she chose divorce. She experienced herself as whirlpooled into hopelessness, feeling unsure and inadequate in her relationship with her husband. She experienced disdain for him as he continued to fall short of her expectations. When she realized the finality of terminating the relationship, she was overwhelmed with the consequences of her choice. Still unsure at the time of the divorce, she experienced intense relief and satisfaction as the overwhelming experience of aloneness and uncertainty was tempered with time.

The data for subject number 2 follow:

Subject #2

Elaborated Description #1

> The most memorable event in my life that involved "sticking with it" was when I decided to go to college for a B.S.N. degree. It was memorable in that I had to really fight for the opportunity to go away to school since my parents, as well as numerous others, were all opposed to the idea. (I think the main thing that it felt like, it was something that I had

really wanted and it felt to me that I was really going out on a limb. It's hard to express. It was like everyone was against me and this was something that I really wanted to accomplish. No matter what I did it didn't seem to be the right thing. A total alienation was what it felt like. Alienation of just everything, and trying to get what I had set out to do.)

Theme #1

When the subject decided to go to college for her B.S.N. degree, she had to really fight for the opportunity as her parents and others were opposed. The subject felt she was really going out on a limb and everyone was against her on something she really wanted to accomplish.

Focal Meaning

For this subject the experience of persisting was struggling for a career she really wanted in the midst of opposition from others.

Elaborated Description #2

I was just out of high school and had not seriously considered what I wanted to do in the future, so I enrolled for a quarter in the local community college. This move was to the absolute delight of my father who taught at the school. While there, I looked into several types of nursing programs. The community college had a two-year program with a one-year waiting list. A local diploma program was three years but I had missed the enrollment date so I would have to wait another year to apply, which would make it four years. Then there was the B.S.N. program that I could transfer easily to since the first year consisted of general study with the following three years containing the nursing courses. The most logical and expedient way for me to be a nurse seemed to be the B.S.N. program.

Theme #2

To the delight of her father, the subject spent a quarter at the local community college where he taught. While there, she looked into several types of nursing programs. The subject believed the most logical and expedient way to be a nurse was the B.S.N. program.

Focal Meaning

The subject complied with her father's educational values when she chose to enroll in a local community college where she ultimately confirmed her career goal.

Elaborated Description #3

When I approached my parents with this idea they were very much opposed. This reaction surprised me and seemed inappropriate and unrealistic since to me, it was such a sound idea. My point was that I could receive the most education for the least amount of time. They could not understand why I would need or want a degree to be a nurse. At that point in time I did not realize the value in obtaining a degree in nursing and what it would mean in the future. I had no knowledge of the entry into practice issue at all. I just felt the B.S.N. program was a better use of my time. My parents presented me with numerous arguments to support their position on the issue. They pointed out all the virtues of being able to live at home and attend school rather than the communal dorm living, having to do my own laundry and quitting my part-time job, etc. They felt my decision was not well thought out and that I just wanted to leave home.

Theme #3

The subject's parents were opposed. This seemed inappropriate and unrealistic and surprised the subject. The subject did not know the value of a nursing degree and just felt the B.S.N. program was a better use of her time. The subject's parents did not understand and presented numerous arguments supporting living at home rather than school. They felt the subject had not thought out her decision well and just wanted to leave home.

Focal Meaning

The subject experienced a clashing of values with parents over her pursuit of a career goal.

Elaborated Description #4

My parents were gaining support for their argument at an alarming rate. (I think the gaining support was definitely for their position. I don't think it was really me trying to move over to them although I did have doubts throughout, you know. I thought—what am I doing?—I really am giving up these certain things that seemed to be okay right now. I think I had a more global view of it or something because they just seemed like they were gaining a lot of support from a lot of different areas where I had never thought that they would look for them. So it was kind of surprising in that way. My father is an accountant for several physicians and being the conscientious accountant and father that he is, he took a survey of the physicians and their nurses to see what type of education was essential to be a nurse. The majority said that a degree, and especially college, was not necessary. One R.N. even told him that if I really wanted to work with people I should be an L.P.N. because R.N.s only do paper work and B.S.N.s only teach.)

Theme #4

The subject's parents were gaining support for their argument from different areas where the subject never thought they would look, which surprised her. The subject had doubts throughout but did not think she was moving over to them. The subject's father was a conscientious accountant and father. He took a survey of physicians for whom he worked and their nurses to see what education was essential to be a nurse. The majority said that a college degree was not necessary.

Focal Meaning

The subject experienced her parents as gaining strength in the clash of differences.

Elaborated Description #5

This was terribly crushing to me, and the more resistance I encountered, the more I wanted to go away to school. (It just seemed like the whole family relationship, specifically of myself to my parents was just being torn apart by this whole thing. Just the fact that they would go around and get other people's opinions about what was happening in a family situation was just kind of—it really made me feel that everywhere I went people would be knowing about this desire, what I had wanted and my parents didn't. Mainly I felt I might be defeated and that was hard. The resistance was more of a pressure kind of feeling. You've just been pushed and pressured into something that you really don't want and the more I felt pressured the more I felt I'd better do something or I'm going to have to take drastic measures or do something. It was that kind of pressure, I felt really trapped and stifled.)

Theme #5

The subject was terribly crushed, and the more resistance she encountered, the more she wanted to go away to school. The subject felt her whole family relationship and specifically that between herself and her parents was being torn apart. The subject was concerned that other people would know what was happening in her family situation—what she wanted and her parents didn't. The subject felt trapped, stifled, pressured, and that she might be defeated which made her feel that she might have to take drastic measures.

Focal Meaning

The subject experienced alienation by being pressured and trapped by her parents' effort to bring about compliance with their values.

Elaborated Description #6

I started to research about nursing education and presented clear documented facts to my parents. I simply had to convince them that I had the ability to make an informed decision.

Theme #6

The subject researched education to present clear documented facts to her parents. The subject had to convince them.

Focal Meaning

The subject felt compelled to confirm her decision-making ability.

Elaborated Description #7

One of the most difficult complicating factors was that they would have to pay for my education. If I went to the community college my tuition would be paid for since my father was employed there. This fact put me in a very precarious position because I needed their financial support for an idea they opposed. (The thing of it was that in order for me to accomplish what I wanted, they would have to finance me. It put me in a position, well, it put them in a situation, too, because they had to agree that, "Yes, we'll send you," because they were financially backing me. If they would have said, "No, we're not going to send you, we're not going to give you the money," then my whole argument would have been up the creek. There would have been no way that I would have gone.)

Theme #7

The subject was in a precarious position because her parents would have to pay tuition, room, and board. If she went to the community college, her tuition would be paid since her father worked there. The subject could not have gone without their financial backing.

Focal Meaning

The subject experienced dissonance while requiring her parents' financial support for something they did not value.

Elaborated Description #8

I feel that some of this opposition was due to a maturational crisis of me leaving home for the first time. Since I am the oldest and the only girl, I think that moving away from the family was particularly stressful. (I think it was stressful for me and the family. I think the stress of me moving away was a breaking away kind of thing. I was real close to my mother, more than any other friends or anything that I'd ever had. That was hard. And it was stressful for them for the same reasons. My mother never worked when we were little. When I went away to school she started to work because she felt she didn't have anything else at home to do. I think it was a particularly hard thing to get used to for everyone within the family and also within myself.) During that time of turmoil I felt very mean and defensive. I felt that my parents thought all I wanted to do was take their money and go away. Even though I felt that way I never gave up the idea of going to school. It was all I talked about and everything I did revolved around that central theme.

Theme #8

The subject was the oldest and the only girl and felt moving away was a maturational crisis which was stressful for herself and her family. The subject was closer to her mother than to friends or anything and the breaking away was hard for all of them. The subject felt very mean and defensive and that her parents thought all she wanted was to take their money and go away. The subject never gave up the idea and everything revolved around that central theme.

Focal Meaning

The subject persisted with her career goal while experiencing the turmoil of a mutual breaking away.

Elaborated Description #9

Finally my parents gave me permission to go [. . .] for one quarter and try it out. It was an unbelievable relief. (It was like, "Oh, I won." I finally got to do what I wanted to do. It was a relief because I felt the relationship between the family was very strained at that time. It just seemed like, "Okay, now I can go, now I can set my thoughts on other things." Because up to that time I was just totally preoccupied with this one goal, this one thing. It was like—now I can really go—it was a relief. Sometimes I thought, "Boy, what if I really mess up, what if this isn't right for me?" Then I kind of got a little scared because I really went out on a limb for this. What if it doesn't work out and I come home defeated, oh. It was a lot of responsibility.)

Theme #9

The subject's parents gave her permission to go for one quarter. The subject felt unbelievable relief and that she had won. The subject felt that she could now set her thoughts on other things. Sometimes the subject was scared that she would mess up, that it wouldn't be right for her and that she had really gone out on a limb and might come home defeated. The subject felt a lot of responsibility.

Focal Meaning

The subject experienced an intermingling of relief and uncertainty as her parents decided to go along with her wishes by placing the responsibility to perform on her.

Elaborated Description #10

The pressure was imposed on me to achieve a 3.0 grade point average or above in each course or else I would have to come home and go to the community college. (I felt that was unnecessary constraint on my being able to go to school but it worked out. But it was very difficult. It did add a lot of pressure. It meant that I had to perform. It put a lot of other constraints on me. If everybody else in the dorm was going out I'd think I'd better not because I have to achieve this. In that kind of way it was more pressure.) Needless to say I did not go home the entire quarter and family relationships were quite strained. (It was just breaking away. It was that I didn't feel comfortable talking to my mother about things that happened at school knowing that she really didn't want me to go there. So when I would be excited about something, I didn't feel I could really share it with my parents because they really didn't want me to be there. That's the way that I felt about it—they really hadn't given me that support to be there so when something good or something bad happened and I needed that support it didn't seem like it was there. So I had to more or less rely on my friends, then. I guess little things—when I first had to go to register I had to go to "drop and add" and it was really a mess. When I told them about it they said, Well, if you'd stayed here you wouldn't have to do that.") I felt I was being punished for a decision I had independently made. As luck would have it I got a 4.0 that quarter and the following one so I was able to stay. (It doesn't feel good. You don't feel too good about yourself. You feel that whatever way you went you're going to get the bad. If you went the other way and stayed home you'd be doing what your parents wanted but you wouldn't be happy with yourself. And then when you go away, you do make this decision and everything's halfway decently okay, then you get this constraint put on you. It didn't feel all that well. It didn't make me feel as though I had made the right decision.)

Theme #10

The pressure to achieve a 3.0 grade point average in each course was imposed, which the subject felt was an unnecessary constraint. This was very difficult as the subject felt that she had to perform and couldn't go out with others in the dorm because of having to achieve this. The subject did not feel comfortable sharing things that happened at school with her parents since they didn't want her to be there. The subject didn't feel she had their support and felt she was being punished for her independent decision. The subject did not feel good about herself. She felt that if she had stayed home as her parents wanted she wouldn't be happy with herself and when she did go away she had the constraints imposed which didn't make her feel she made the right decision.

Focal Meaning

The subject experienced disdain in the unreasonable constraints placed on her by her parents even though her performance complied with their demands.

Elaborated Description #11

Four years later when I graduated my father told me that he thought I had made a good decision and apologized for giving me such a hard time. He stated that he did not trust my judgment at that time but realized now that I had accomplished something that was very important to me. It was only then that I felt truly good about my decision. My satisfaction with myself for making a decision, fighting for the right to accomplish what I had decided to do, and then to be told that I had made the right decision by those who had opposed me, was very self-gratifying. (It was really nice to know that my father, especially, had come back and said that I did make a good decision. That made me feel as though I really made this decision and I went through with it even though there was so much resistance. I came out and it was good. And then, they know it was good. And so that even made it all that much better because I knew within myself that it was a good choice and it all worked out okay. Then to have somebody else who was the main opposer to say, "Hey, you did all right." That was a good thing. Then you think, "Wow, I really did do that" and that was really like the icing on the cake. It was really nice. And we joke about it now. It was a really good feeling. And then he asked me, "Well, aren't you going to go and get your master's degree?" I said, "Are you kidding me?" That was the best, it was a really gratifying situation. It made me feel very happy.)

Theme #11

When the subject graduated, her father apologized for giving her a hard time and said she made a good decision. The subject's father realized that she had accomplished something very important to her. The subject then felt truly good about her decision, satisfied and self-gratified. The subject knew within herself that it was a good choice and to have her main opposer say, "I'm glad you did that," was the icing on the cake. The subject's father asked her if she was going to get her master's degree—and she was very happy.

Focal Meaning

At the time of graduation, the subject experienced satisfaction in the success of her persisting in the face of opposition when confirmed by her parents who had opposed her.

The focal meanings were synthesized into a situated structural description for subject number 2. The situated structural definition follows:

Situated Structural Description #2

For this subject in this situation, the experience of persisting even though it is difficult was struggling for a career she wanted as her parents opposed her. She complied with her father's educational values when she enrolled in the local community college where he taught. But while there she ultimately confirmed her career goal of attaining a bachelor of science degree at a university. She experienced a clashing of values with her parents over her choice of this goal. She experienced alienation as she was pressured and felt trapped by her parents' efforts to convince her to stay and comply with their values. She experienced dissonance as she required her parents' support for her goal which they did not value. She needed their financial support. She was the first child to want to leave home. As she persisted with her goal, she and her family experienced the turmoil of a mutual breaking away.

She experienced an intermingling of relief and uncertainty as her parents decided to go along with her wishes but placed on her the responsibility of performing at a 3.0 grade point level. She experienced disdain in the unreasonable constraints placed on her by her parents even though her performance complied with their demands.

At the time of graduation, she experienced much satisfaction in the success of her persisting in the face of opposition—as her choice was now confirmed by her parents who had opposed her.

After dwelling with the two situated structural descriptions, the essences of each were synthesized into a general structural description which reflects the meaning of the phenomenon as it emerged from the lived experiences of both subjects.

General Structural Description

The experience of *persisting even though it is difficult* emerges in the pushing-resisting of close interhuman relationships where there are conflicting values. The individual experiences turmoil in the ambiguity and conflict of the situation in which there is a certain feeling of being bound or trapped. As the individual chooses anew from among possible alternatives, the struggle to stay with that choice unfolds.

In the powering that is lived in the choosing of the valued alternatives and persisting with that choice even though it is difficult, the individual lives a rhythmical pattern of certainty-uncertainty, experiences feelings of aloneness and helplessness and of being sure of the rightness of the choice all at once. The individual experiences disdain and dissonance as the struggle to persist is lived.

In *persisting even though it is difficult* there is an expansion of the boundaries of the interhuman relationship as the individual experiences relief and ultimate satisfaction and the new value is affirmed. A growing satisfaction with self emerges as the persisting situation is distanced over time.

DISCUSSION OF FINDINGS

The findings which emerge from this phenomenological study will be discussed in relation to the data and the researcher's perspective of the phenomenon.

Persisting even though it is difficult is expressed in patterns of pushing-resisting in close interhuman relationships where values conflict. For each subject, patterns of pushing-resisting were lived in relation to values that conflicted with those of the close other. For the first subject, pushing-resisting is seen in the marital relationship as the subject began to value dissolving the relationship and her husband valued staying with the relationship. For the second subject, pushing-resisting emerged as the subject valued a baccalaureate degree education which involved leaving home, while her parents valued an associate degree education which would involve staying at home. As discussed in the section of this study on researcher's perspective, (Parse, 1981) describes the pushing-resisting of every encounter as a reflection of the powering inherent in the struggle and conflict in the situation (pp. 57-59). The subjects, then, experienced pushing-resisting as they lived the clash of powering in their encounters with their close others as their valuing conflicted and new possibilities were illuminated, considered, and embraced. It is in this risking to persist even though it is difficult that the pushing-resisting tension and emerging conflict were lived. Subjects chose to stay with the struggle in light of their valued goals and the ambiguity of the unknown outcomes.

Turmoil is experienced in the ambiguity and conflict of the binding situation from the struggle of *persisting in change even though it is difficult*. Each subject experienced turmoil as the conflict, with its inherent ambiguous outcomes, was confronted. The first subject experienced turmoil with the choice of divorce in the face of clashing perspectives of husband and family and friends. The subject did not know the outcome—whether it would be better or worse—and the experience of turmoil surfaced within the situation. The second subject's experience of turmoil emerged as the subject persisted in her career goal and the family experienced a mutual breaking away. The subject was caught within the conflict of her own goal and that of her parents. Persisting in her own goal meant leaving home and family against their wishes and with no guarantee of success. In choosing and staying with her goal, the subject was both enabled and limited. "In this choosing, Man enables self to move in one direction and limits movement in another" (Parse 1981, p. 53). Turmoil emerges, then, as an experience inherent in the enabling-limiting of choosing and affirming a valued alternative in spite of difficulty and ambiguity.

There is a rhythmical pattern of certainty-uncertainty (Parse, pp. 60-61) as the struggle to affirm the valued alternative unfolds. For the first subject, the rhythm of certainty-uncertainty unfolded as she considered the alternatives—staying with her husband who still loved her but did not meet her expectations, or divorcing him in quest of what might be. The subject describes being sure and unsure, a "wavering." For the second subject, also, the pattern of certainty-uncertainty emerges in the consideration and choice of alternatives. The subject was certain of her career goal in the face of opposition and the unknown outcome and yet was also uncertain—"What if I really mess up, what if this isn't right for me?" For each subject the experience of certainty-uncertainty was an all-at-once rhythmical pattern. In making the choice to persist in spite of difficulty, the subjects considered and affirmed their valued alternatives while simultaneously giving up what was, as well as possibilities other than those chosen. As the subjects persisted in their choosing of the valued alternative, they lived choosing and rechoosing as the rhythmical pattern of certainty-uncertainty surfaced in the struggle of staying with the valued goal.

Inherent in the experience of *persisting even though it is difficult* are feelings of aloneness, helplessness, disdain, sureness, and rightness, which reflect the unity of persisting in a difficult situation. For each subject these feelings unfolded as they lived the rhythmical pattern of certainty-uncertainty. The first subject experienced uncertainty—feeling alone, helpless, and unsure. When she was with her husband she was not understood and experienced disdain as her expectations were not met. She experienced sureness and a feeling of rightness as the certainty in this certainty-uncertainty unity surfaced when the choosing of divorce became the valued alternative. Similarly, the second subject experienced feelings of uncertainty—of aloneness, helplessness, and unsureness—as she considered her goal in the face of the opposition of her loved parents. She experienced sureness and knowing that her goal was right in light of her investigation into the values of a baccalaureate nursing education and her valuing of the choice. She experienced disdain for her parents as they added constraints as a condition for allowing her to proceed toward her goal. Thus, the experiences of aloneness, helplessness, disdain, sureness, and rightness are interwoven in the certainty-uncertainty rhythm which unfolds in the powering of the enabling-limiting of valuing that is persisting in a difficult situation.

Persisting even though it is difficult involves an expansion of the boundaries of the interhuman relationship. For the first subject, the choosing of divorce severed the bonds of the marital contract, thus enabling the scope of the interhuman relationship to be broadened. Each spouse was freed from the limits of marriage and thus free to bring other individuals into close relationship and so to move further from one another. The second subject, in choosing to leave home to engage in the educational process, also experienced an expansion of the interhuman boundaries. Including new acquaintances and friends served to broaden the bounds of the interpersonal scope of the family. In this sharing of the interhuman relationship with others there is also a broadening of the meanings cocreated in family as new perspectives are shared. In this persistence in the choice of divorce and of baccalaureate education, the subjects enabled movement in one direction—the expansion of interpersonal boundaries—and limited movement in another (Parse, 1981, p. 53).

Relief and satisfaction emerge as the persisting situation is distanced over time. The subjects experienced relief as goals were reached and distanced. For the first subject, the experience of uncertainty was still present at the divorce proceedings. The subject described relief and satisfaction surfacing a week after the divorce. For the second subject, also, the experience of uncertainty remained as she was given permission to pursue her baccalaureate education. Relief emerged in the light of her parents' decision to allow her to go and the struggle to convince them was distanced. For this subject, satisfaction emerged at the time of graduation—four years from the time of the decision. As described in the section of this study on the researcher's perspective, van Kaam (1972) writes, ". . . it is not enough to know what road I should take among the many possible roads offered to me. I must walk that road and keep walking" (pp. 4-5). For these subjects, then, the experience of relief and satisfaction emerged as they "kept walking"—as the persisting situation was distanced over time.

The description of the lived experience which emerged from the findings of this study follows:

> The experience of persisting even though it is difficult involves living paradoxical patterns of relating which embody turmoil, emerging relief, and satisfaction as growth is enhanced.

While each subject described unrelated life experiences in answering the question posed, many similarities in the lived experience emerged. These have been related to the researcher's perspective in the discussion of the findings. The results of the study indicate congruence of the lived experience (as elaborated in the two descriptions), with the nursing theory, Man-Living-Health (Parse, 1981).

Living paradoxical patterns of relating points to the principle that "cocreating rhythmical patterns of relating is living the paradoxical unity of revealing-concealing and enabling-limiting while connecting-separating." (Parse, 1981) It was evident in the descriptions by subjects that they experienced paradoxes and expressed being enabled-limited by the choices they made to persist in a difficult situation. While they each chose to move in one direction, which enabled independence, against the wishes of another, the husband for subject 1 and the father for subject 2, their independence was simultaneously limited by the views others had of them. Experiencing turmoil and emerging relief and satisfaction relates directly to the principle "structuring meaning multidimensionally is cocreating reality through the languaging of valuing and imaging" (Parse, 1981). Turmoil was the meaning given to the ambiguous situation both subjects described. Choosing to live the turmoil by persisting reflects a valuing of self. This valuing gave rise to the emerging relief and satisfaction which was the meaning the subjects gave to the experience.

The idea that growth is enhanced through persisting relates to the principle, "cotranscending with the possibles is powering unique ways of originating in the process of transforming" (Parse, 1981). Enhancing growth is a way of powering toward what is not-yet. Growing is changing toward diversity and complexity, reflecting the pushing-resisting through interhuman relationships in the experience of persisting even though it is difficult.

In light of the correspondence of the principles of Man-Living-Health with the general structural description of the lived experience of persisting even though it is difficult, the theory of Man-Living-Health is supported.

VI

THE ETHNOGRAPHIC METHOD

E thnography is defined as the branch of anthropology that concerns itself with scientific descriptions of cultural groups. It is a research method aimed at uncovering order in the voluminous data gathered through participant observation and informant inquiry. The researcher enters the world of the participants and explores with them the symbols, rituals, and customs of their world. Through an exhaustive process of observing, discussing, questioning, and validating, the researcher enlarges personal knowledge of the particular culture and records the world of others as they conceptualize it. In a classic paper, Sturtevant (1966) quotes Malinowski on this point:

> The final goal, of which an Ethnographer should never lose sight . . . is, briefly, to grasp the native's point of view, his relation to life, to realize *his* vision of *his* world (p. 476).

This directive from the early 1920's is as significant today as it was then and, as the procedures of the method continue to be refined, this original aim persists. In coming to understand the ethnographic method, it is important to consider the continuing dialogue between the proponents of the two approaches called *emic* and *etic*. Both approaches have their roots in linguistics.

The *emic* approach is related to the semantics or meanings inherent in cultural organization of knowledge. In this approach, the conceptualizations of a particular group must be studied and categorized in the language of the "insider's" view. This approach is designed to examine how the various elements of a particular group unfold in relationship to each other (Pelto and Pelto, p. 54). Frake (1964), in his discussion of approach, emphasizes the importance of the "insider's" view in this way:

The test of descriptive adequacy must always refer to informants' interpretation of events, not simply to the occurrence of events (p. 112).

The *etic* approach points precisely to this "occurrence of events." Harris (1968) describes the etic approach as one in which:

> . . . the phenomenal distinctions are judged appropriate by the community of scientific observers . . . etic statements are verified when independent observers using similar operations agree that a given event has occurred (p. 575).

The etic or "outsider's" view would use quantitative analysis of patterns of behavior as defined by the observer (Pelto and Pelto, p. 62).

Although the controversy over the merits of each approach continues, Pelto and Pelto propose that "the once clear differences between emic and etic assumptions are somewhat blurred" (p. 65). They suggest that researchers frequently use "combinations of emic and etic data" (p. 65). Both approaches, then, serve the research effort well when used appropriately to the question under study and the theoretical perspective of the researcher.

PURPOSE

All ethnographic studies have a broad, general purpose, which is to come to understand the cultural meanings people use to organize and interpret their experiences (Spradley, 1979, p. 93). This general purpose gives direction to the particular culture chosen for study in light of the researcher's interest.

It is characteristic of the ethnographic method that the purpose may shift as the study evolves. For example, Becker, et al. (1961), in their classic study of medical students, began their investigation with the purpose of exploring medical school as an organization where students acquired perspectives on their later activities as doctors. However, as they analyzed their data, they noticed that a different focus emerged, which they called the "level and direction of academic effort" (pp. 419-423). It was this shift that became the focused purpose of the study.

The ethnographic method, like other qualitative and quantitative methods, is a research approach encompassing five basic elements: 1. identifying the phenomenon; 2. structuring the study; 3. gathering the data; 4. analyzing the data; and 5. describing the findings.

IDENTIFYING THE PHENOMENON

The phenomenon in the ethnographic study is a question that is researchable through coming to understand the meanings of symbolic patterns that unfold in the structure of language. For example, phenomena worthy of study might be the experience of play for preschoolers or the experience of celebration for graduating seniors.

STRUCTURING THE STUDY

The second element in the ethnographic method is structuring the study plan. This includes specifying a research question which makes explicit the researcher's intent in studying a particular phenomenon, clarifying the researcher's perspective of the phenomenon, identifying a study sample, and protecting the rights of subjects.

The Research Question

Research questions, such as, "How do kindergarten children language the meaning of play?" or "How do graduating seniors language the celebration of the event?" and "How do persons with cancer express the meaning of their pain?" may be studied by the ethnographic method. These questions are congruent with the nursing perspective presented in Chapter II of this text, and guide the formulation of the data-gathering statement which leads to the uncovering of the phenomenon.

Researcher's Perspective

The researcher's beliefs about the phenomenon are made explicit in the ethnographic method. The perspective is a frame of reference which is identified early in the study. The ethnographer *brackets* personal bias so as to come to know the daily life of individuals as they live it. To bracket means to make the researcher's perspective explicit through parenthetical inclusion, and to hold that perspective in abeyance when approaching the data for analysis and synthesis.

Study Sample

The sample consists of a culture group which is living the phenomenon under study. Any group of people who share knowledge, customs, objects, events, and activities is considered a culture (Spradley, p. 6). In light of this broad definition of culture, any group of people may be chosen for a study, depending on the researcher's interests. The number of subjects is not particularly relevant to the ethnographic method. Selected from the group are *key informants* and *general informants*, who can share information and knowledge about the phenomenon under study as they are living it.

Protecting the Rights of Human Subjects

Because of the nature of ethnographic studies, it is possible in many situations to study unobtrusively and, therefore, without permission. Spradley (1980) identifies three types of social situations with regard to permission. The first is the "free entry" setting, such as a public place, where research can be done without permission. The second is the "limited entry" setting (e.g., offices, schools, hospitals, and treatment centers) where permission is required of one or more persons. The third is the "restricted entry" setting, which is exemplified by closed meetings and secret societies (pp. 49-50). Subjects' rights are protected by obtaining appropriate permission and by assuring anonymity in reporting results. The purpose of the study is explained to participants and is repeated in many ways in order to develop the questioning-dialoguing that occurs throughout the study. Key informants are apprised of their option to withdraw at any time throughout the study. General informants are apprised of their right not to talk with the researcher.

DATA GATHERING

This phase begins with general observations and questions which are recorded as the beginning ethnographic record. The ethnographic record consists of "field notes, tape recordings, pictures, artifacts, and anything else which documents the culture scene under study" (Spradley, 1979, p. 69). This is the main body of evidence which is expanded through several levels of ethnographic inquiry and ethnographic analysis as the study progresses.

The major processes through which ethnographic research unfolds are participant observation and ethnographic interview.

Participant observation is a way of involved watching. Because of the special nature of this involvement, participant observation can be considered a way of being present in which the researcher transcends ordinary participation in a group. Spradley (1980) distinguishes between the "ordinary participant" in a setting and the participant observer. The ordinary observer generally participates in a setting for the purpose of engaging in the daily activities. The participant observer not only engages in the activities but also watches all aspects of the situation for the purpose of recording and analyzing the happenings (p. 56). The involved "watcher" of the situation is one who becomes . . . explicitly aware of things that others take for granted" (Spradley, 1979, p. 58). In a sense, Spradley (1979) proposes that the spirit of the emic and etic approaches are engaged simultaneously in the process of participant observation. He describes this as both the "insider and outsider" perspective inherent in the process of participant observation.

Ethnographic inquiry is the companion process to participant-observation and is "used to best advantage when it is closely integrated with participant observation" (Pelto and Pelto, 1981, p. 74). Because of the close relationship of the researcher to the culture under study, there is an advantage to the trust that surfaces between them. It is this close relationship, however, that "may significantly color the information given by the informant" (Pelto and Pelto, 1981, p. 74). Much controversy surrounds this process of ethnographic inquiry for many reasons: bias, incomplete knowledge, a possible tendency to tell the researcher what the researcher wants to hear and, certainly not least among the criticisms, the unstructured talking and "hanging around." Spradley (1979) attempts to put some of these criticisms to rest in his description of the ethnographic interview as a "particular kind of speech event which is identified by a special kind of talking" (p. 55). He identifies the elements of the ethnographic interview as "explicit purpose, ethnographic explanations and ethnographic questions" (p. 59).

Ethnographic inquiry, then, is a complex way of interrelating with informants which includes appropriately informal conversation and deliberate, focused questioning designed to elicit rich cultural meanings. Ethnographic inquiry involves interviewing key people in a group as well as the informal interviewing of many persons in the situation.

Spradley (1979) has identified three major types of questions that are helpful as interviewing strategies.

DESCRIPTIVE QUESTIONS (those which elicit a word picture of the way persons represent their world to themselves) are designed to expand the explanations of participants and are used throughout the different phases of the study. Spradley (1979) says that descriptive questions "form the backbone of all ethnographic interviews" (p. 91). Some examples of descriptive questions are:

Tell me what you did yesterday from the time you got up until you went to bed.

Tell me what happens when you go to current events.

STRUCTURAL QUESTIONS are those which seek to understand not only *what* people know but *how* they organize what they know (Spradley, 1979, p. 131). Structural questions both complement and expand descriptive data as they uncover the systematic organization of the culture. Some examples of structural questions are:

We've been talking about the different kinds of activities that take place in a nursing home. I'm interested in getting a list of all the different kinds of activities or at least all the ones you do—could you tell me some?

Are there different ways to pass the time in a nursing home?

What are the ways in which nurses do things for you?

CONTRAST QUESTIONS are designed to compare in order to show differences. Symbols in a meaning system are related to each other by both their similarities and their differences. Contrast questions focus on how symbols differ from each other (Spradley, 1979, p. 157). They are formulated as the researcher notes particular differences in the way an informant describes the symbols in conversation. Some examples of contrast questions are:

We've been talking about "ways to get through the day" and in going over our talks, there are some differences I'd like to ask you about. You mentioned "casual talking with your roommate" and "talking with friends or relatives"—would you say these are different because visitors can tell you about the "outside" and your roommate cannot?

Would you say that dying "in here" is different from dying "out there" because "in here" there is nothing to do but "the waiting" to die?

These three types of questions and their many subtypes identified by Spradley (1979, p. 223) are suggested for facilitating the collection of rich cultural data that will expand and verify the ethnographic record. While all questions are appropriate in all studies, they are not used sequentially nor are they all used to the same extent. These categories are suggested as guidelines to be used in a synthetic way as the researcher becomes more skilled in the ethnographic method.

DATA ANALYSIS

Collection and analysis of data can best be described as a simultaneous process that occurs in a spiral of increasing complexity rather than along a linear continuum. Table 7 shows this spiral. In other words, the researcher does not proceed from predetermined hypotheses to conclusions, but rather through levels of collection and analysis of data. As one ascends through the various levels in the spiral, new dimensions of understanding are uncovered and new questions emerge which expand and verify the findings. This phase proceeds simultaneously with data collection through several levels as the researcher seeks out the meaning of the cultural symbols inherent in informants' language.

Domain Analysis

The first level of analysis begins from the ethnographic record of general observations and questioning. An initial domain search for simple naming yields tentative domains to be expanded and hypothetical propositions to be tested with the participants. A domain is a symbolic category which includes other smaller categories. The first level of analysis proceeds from this initial search for domains to a domain analysis as it seeks to uncover semantic relationships among the terms used over and above the simple names. This first level of analysis uncovers relational patterns which help the researcher to formulate structural and additional descriptive questions in the next phase of data gathering. These relational patterns are then categorized according to a linguistic framework. The most commonly used framework is the *universal semantic relationship framework*, which represents the type of semantic relationships believed to be present in all cultures. Some of these universal semantic relationships are spatial, strict inclusion, attribution, means-end, and rationale (Spradley, 1979).

Taxonomic Analysis

The next level of analysis, the taxonomic, is the point at which the researcher must choose how the study will continue. The choice is to proceed with a surface analysis which investigates as many domains as possible, or to focus on an in-depth study of only a few domains. Obviously, there is controversy about the relative merits of

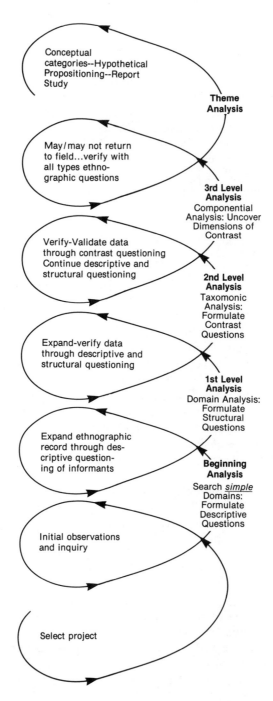

Conceptual
categories--Hypothetical
Propositioning--Report
Study

**Theme
Analysis**

May/may not return
to field...verify with
all types ethno-
graphic questions

**3rd Level
Analysis**
Componential
Analysis: Uncover
Dimensions of
Contrast

Verify-Validate data
through contrast questioning
Continue descriptive and
structural questioning

**2nd Level
Analysis**
Taxomonic
Analysis:
Formulate
Contrast
Questions

Expand-verify data
through descriptive and
structural questioning

**1st Level
Analysis**
Domain Analysis:
Formulate
Structural
Questions

Expand ethnographic
record through des-
criptive question-
ing of informants

**Beginning
Analysis**

Search *simple*
Domains:
Formulate
Descriptive
Questions

Initial observations
and inquiry

Select project

TABLE 7   COLLECTION AND ANALYSIS OF DATA SPIRAL

each. A compromise frequently made is the selection of a few domains for in-depth analysis and the others for an "holistic perspective of the whole culture" (Spradley, 1979, p. 134). Whichever procedure is selected, the taxonomic level of analysis is directed toward uncovering a single semantic relationship within a domain; that is, a taxonomy demonstrates the internal organization of a domain. As the researcher progresses in the taxonomic analysis, ethnographic inquiry is alternated with participant-observation to validate the taxonomy. It is important to remember that taxonomies always approximate the way a culture "organizes its knowledge" (Spradley, 1979, p. 150) and that eventually the collecting, analyzing, and verifying of data must end. Spradley (1979) makes it quite clear, "ultimately, the ethnographer makes the decision about how to represent the data . . . in ways that go beyond the data" (p. 150).

The domain and taxonomic analyses, then, examine single semantic relationships, focusing on units of organization and the relationship among the subsets of the unit.

Componential Analysis

The third level of analysis, componential, studies multiple relationships by examining components of meaning. Components of meaning are the attributes that surface in relation to differences rather than similarities among the categories of each domain. Again, the researcher analyzes the data for contrasts among the categories and designs contrast questions that will validate the analysis with the participants. In this process, additional semantic relationships that do not seem to cohere with the taxonomy may be revealed.

Theme Analysis

The final level in the analysis of data is uncovering cultural themes. Cultural themes are conceptualizations that connect domains, giving a holistic view of the culture under study. Themes are best uncovered in a process Spradley (1979) calls immersion. This means that the researcher deeply engages with the culture, expanding and testing the ethnographic record. This occurs through intensive dwelling with the data and subsequent verification with the subjects.

The recurring themes lead the researcher to the generation of conceptualizations and their identifying properties. It is important to remember that, although the grounding of the observations is in the world of the participants, the data are always screened through the filter of the researcher's method. The generation of conceptualizations represents a transformational shift in the level of abstraction within the content of the discipline.

The data are then synthesized into hypothetical propositions. These propositions reflect the data rooted in the participants' reality and synthesized within the researcher's method. They represent the researcher's conceptualization about the culture studied.

DESCRIBING THE FINDINGS

Describing the findings of an ethnographic study requires the presentation of the hypothetical propositions as they emerged from the analysis. Because of the large quantity of data, only examples are shown in the report of ethnographic studies. A discussion is included with the description of findings which relates the hypothetical propositions to the frame of reference.

The next chapter explicitly demonstrates the implementation of the ethnographic method.

VII

THE EXPERIENCE OF AGING
AN ETHNOGRAPHIC STUDY

PURPOSE

The purpose of this study was to generate hypothetical propositions about the ways in which the elderly interpret their world in a
variety of settings. The rationale for choosing the ethnographic
method for this study was that it is directed toward uncovering the
perspective of a phenomenon as it is being lived by the subjects being
studied. It is a human science method in which the researcher participates with the subject group in search of what it is like to live a
particular experience.

RESEARCH QUESTION

The research question guiding this study was: What is the
meaning of aging among the elderly in a variety of settings?

PHENOMENON

The phenomenon central to this study is the experience of aging. Many theories, following the pattern of Erik Erikson's (1963) "8
stages of man" are based on chronological phases through which one
passes. In the journey through life's chronology, persons must successfully complete the tasks of one stage before embracing the next
one. Although the authors emphasize that the stages are not inexora-
ble and that individuals do not necessarily conform to them in a

rigid, sequential order, there is at least a tacit suggestion that the tasks of earlier stages must be successfully negotiated before moving to the next stage. It is characteristic of the "stage" theorists that the work is rooted in a perspective of hierarchical linearity.

Theories that do not propose hierarchical stages are beginning to emerge. For example, Katchadourian (1978) illuminates the cultural and historical influence that must be considered and Neugarten (1973) emphasizes the importance of context in the study of aging. "The condition of the aged depends upon the social context . . . it is the meaning that men attribute to their life, it is their entire system of values that defines the meaning and value of old age" (p. 131). In light of this, aging can only be "understood as a whole."

Rogers (1970) suggests a view of aging consistent with the focus of nursing as the science of unitary man. For her, aging is a creative process that continues throughout life as man grows in diversity and complexity. She does not focus on diseases in aging, and in fact says that "aging is not a disease . . . that health and illness are a part of the same phenomenon and that . . . events taking place in one's life axis are expressions of health" (p. 125). Parse (1981) proposes that "health is a continuously changing process that man participates in cocreating" (p. 41).

Researcher's Perspective

The researcher's perspective of the experience of aging is consistent with the views of Rogers (1970) and Parse (1981). The researcher's perspective of aging is that it is one's journey toward increasingly complex configurations of the whole in the ascent into personal death. This means that as one moves toward the reality of non-being one generates new awarenesses which lead to a renewed commitment to a purpose in life. This commitment to purpose guides the reordering of priorities, which creates a shifting of views of cherished values and imagined possibles.

Sample

The sample in this study consisted of older adults in three nursing homes. One key informant was identified in each of two of these three nursing homes. There were also subjects from two multipurpose centers, one day care center for aged persons, and several individual family homes.

PROTECTION OF SUBJECTS' RIGHTS

Protection of human subjects was accomplished by assuring anonymity and explaining the nature of subject participation. Their right to choose not to participate or to cease participation at any time was carefully explained to subjects in a variety of ways. Special care was taken to ensure that the elderly subjects understood the nature of their participation. The researcher met with administrators and directors of nursing to explain the purpose of the study. In one nursing home, the researcher also attended "family night" to explain the project to residents and their families. Anyone who wished not to participate was not approached; it is interesting to note that, in one nursing home where four persons declined to participate, three later changed their minds and joined the researcher in informal discussions.

DATA GATHERING

Data were gathered through informal conversations with many residents, ethnographic interviews with the two key informants, and participant-observation in all settings. The period of study continued for eight months, with the most intensive observations occurring in the first four months. In these first four months, observations took place three times a week, averaging in length from three to six hours each day between 9:00 a.m. and 8:00 p.m. Three observations took place between 10:00 p.m. and 6:00 a.m. In this way, the researcher was present at the research scene over a broad spectrum of time. The ethnographic record was reviewed for domains, which are the symbolic categories that include other categories. This initial search was directed toward seeking simple naming of things by informants. After identification of these simple domains, the researcher returned to the informants to validate and expand the ethnographic record in preparation for the first level of analysis. Then, the researcher returned to the informants at the successive levels of analysis in order to verify data gathered and further expand the ethnographic record.

DATA ANALYSIS

Data analysis was simultaneous with data gathering throughout the life of the study. The domain analysis began as the expanded ethnographic record was examined for semantic relationships. These relational patterns guided the researcher in formulating structural questions which served to further expand the data at the next level of ethnographic inquiry and guide participant-observation. Through structural and descriptive questioning, the domains were validated and again expanded in preparation for the second level of analysis, the taxonomic.

The taxonomic analysis was initiated by the researcher's choice to select a few domains for in-depth analysis and to continue a surface examination of others. The surface focus on all domains with in-depth analysis of only a few offered both a perspective of the culture as a whole and a deeper understanding of the chosen domains. Domains were chosen for an in-depth analysis by the researcher for two reasons. One was theoretical interest related to how aged persons live their health and another was related to the principle of organizing domains. An organizing domain is one that appears to structure many other domains. Five domains were chosen which seemed to include some elements of most of the remaining domains, thus creating an organizing principle among all the domains. For the in-depth analysis of the selected domains, field notes were carefully examined for possible relationships among all terms in the domain and tentative taxonomies were constructed. Taxonomies were analyzed for relationships and contrast questions were formulated. These contrast questions, as well as additional structural and descriptive questions, formed the basis for the data gathering in the subsequent ethnographic interviews and participant-observation.

In componential analysis, the researcher examined the categories of meaning related to the similarities as well as to the differences among the categories. This third level of analysis also identified additional relationships in informant comments that did not seem to cohere with the taxonomies, yet yielded profound insights into the meaning of aging for the informants. Componential analysis marked the completion of regularly scheduled ethnographic interviews and participant-observation. Periodically throughout the remaining phases of the study, the researcher returned to the informants to share the unfolding conceptualizations.

Major and minor themes were uncovered in the theme analysis as the researcher became immersed in the ethnographic record. Testing and validating of the themes with participants occurred at the researcher's discretion. Eventually, collecting, analyzing and verifying must end and this analysis of data for recurring themes signaled the final level of analysis for this study. The last two phases of the study shifted to a focus on synthesis and creative conceptualization in the researcher's representation of the data. The researcher engaged in a profound dwelling with the major and minor themes. In this intensive process, the researcher was immersed in reliving the long engagement with the whole study. The conceptual categories represent the tacit and explicit understandings of the researcher, framed within the transformational shifts toward concepts of a higher order in the ladder of abstraction.

The conceptual categories and their identifying properties were then synthesized into hypothetical propositions which reflect a description of the phenomenon of aging interpreted by selected informants and synthesized by the researcher. They are provisional hypotheses that could be used to design further investigation of this phenomenon.

Presentation of Data

The model used for the presentation of data was derived from Spradley (1979). The domain analysis, which is the first level of analysis, yielded 18 domains representing seven different universal semantic relationships (see Appendix B1). Five of these domains were selected for in-depth analysis and the remainder were pursued at the surface level. The five domains chosen for in-depth analysis were:

1. Ways to get through the day,
2. Kinds of problems,
3. Kinds of relationships,
4. Ways to create privacy,
5. Kinds of fears.

The domains and their included terms are in the language of the informant and they are presented in Appendix B2.

In the second level of analysis, the taxonomic, the five domains were examined for subsets of the semantic relationship identified, and a taxonomy was generated for each of the five domains analyzed in-depth. As an example, the taxonomy for the domain, "Ways to Get Through the Day," appears in Appendix B3.

The purpose of the third level of analysis, the componential, is to uncover the components of meaning within a system. This was done by examining the ethnographic record for contrasts in meaning among the informants' language symbols. Segments of two field notes demonstrating this, taken from the ethnographic record in the taxonomy for the domain "Ways to Get Through the Day," follow:

1. Attribute: Casual Talking

Talking with visitors is different from talking with roommates because roommates can only talk about what's going on in here—and then, Honey, talking with nurses is different, too. You have to be careful when you talk to the nurses, honey, see—she's the boss—if you make them mad at you—well—they just say you're agitated—or, ok, what's that other word—yes—yes—combative, that's it—they give you medicine—they put it in your food, you know, honey—look at (N)—they put sedatives in her food—sometimes you can see it—little white powder—I just don't eat it—I pretend I'm not hungry—you have to be careful.

2. Attribute: Waiting to Die:

It's not so bad knowing you're soon going to die—at my age and with all my problems—I'm ready—but in here—see, when I was in my own place—I didn't just wait for death to come and get me—I went out a little—had my friends to tea—oh, I did things—in here—you just wait—you wait—to die.

These two examples from the field notes show that there are differences in casual talking with roommates and with nurses and in waiting to die "in here." All field notes were reviewed for such differences and the following are two examples of contrast statements framed by the researcher emerging from the taxonomy for the domain, "Ways to Get Through the Day":

1. Attribute: Casual Talking

Casual talking with nurses is different from casual talking with your roommate, because the nurse is "the boss."

2. Attribute: "Waiting to Die"

Waiting to die "in here" is different from knowing you're going to die when you're out there because here—there's *nothing* but to wait for it.

An inventory of such contrast statements was prepared and validated with informants through contrast questioning as well as through additional structural and descriptive questioning. The dimensions of contrast evolving from this analysis for the domain "Ways to Get Through the Day" are:

1. Things you can control,
2. Things you have to be careful about,

3. Things that hold some degree of interest,

4. Things that make you feel cared about.

A sample of the componential analysis for selected subsets of the domain, "Ways to Get Through the Day," appears in Appendix B4. The componential analysis also provides another form of information in the search for contrasts. As the researcher guides the informants to elaborate the interview data, additional relationships surface that do not seem connected to the taxonomies. For example, "pretending you're still in your own home" was an attribute of the taxonomy: "Ways to Get Through the Day." The following structural question was asked to elaborate this attribute:

Question:

What are all the things you can think of that *pretending you're still at home* does to help you get through the day?

Informant response:

Pretending you're still at home keeps you from thinking about your family putting you here—not wanting you—it makes it easier to get through the day because—you can be happy—and maybe—not so mad—you pretend you're a young woman again—getting the supper ready—you're not so lonesome—if you can remember all that—well— maybe—maybe you won't go—senile.

In analyzing this segment of field notes, relationships were uncovered that did not cohere with the taxonomy. An example of these additional relationships for "pretending you're still at home" appears in Table 8.

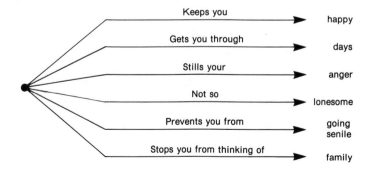

TABLE 8 ADDITIONAL RELATIONSHIPS

These additional relationships complement the growing body of data and enhance the researcher's understanding of the informants' world as they conceptualize it. All of these additional relationships were reviewed as the researcher dwelled with the data in the final phases of the study.

The fourth level of analysis is the search for themes. Four major themes and associated minor themes surfaced as the ethnographic record was reviewed again. These themes are:

1. Pervading sense of surrender of one's self to the system;
   a. Recurring attempts to please staff,
   b. Hesitance to ask for help unless absolutely necessary,
   c. Increasing acceptance of lack of privacy,
   d. Increasing immunity to staff neglect and borderline cruelty,
   e. Conspicuous absence of asserting one's self-reliance.

2. Curiosity about and interest in the topic of death;
   a. Growing realization that life was nearing the end,
   b. Quiet gratitude for a long, good life in spite of all obstacles,
   c. Expectant hope for a peaceful and dignified death,
   d. Repeated statement of the desire not to become a burden to anyone,
   e. Anxious fear of dying and not being discovered until morning,
   f. Repeated wish not to prolong death with mechanical-technical assistance,
   g. Speculative questioning about what comes after death.

3. Growing acceptance of meaningless time;
   a. Open willingness to participate in boring activities just to pass the day,
   b. Increasing contentment to sit in front of television sets,
   c. Going through the motions just to please the staff,
   d. Docile acceptance of incessant waiting,
   e. Unquestioning acceptance of staff directives, instructions, and mixed messages.

4. Dreadful images of the nursing home as a place to wait for death;
   a. Haunting sense of suspended waiting,
   b. An unspoken directive to put your "best foot forward,"
   c. An abiding sense of being "on your best behavior."
   d. A pervasive ambiance of suffocating politeness.

Once the themes were identified and the ethnographic record was reviewed once again in its entirety, the conceptual categories and hypothetical propositions were generated by the researcher. The conceptual categories, with some of their identifying properties and the hypothetical propositions, are presented in Table 9. Each proposition, with one supporting field note from each of the settings, appears in Appendix B5.

DISCUSSION OF FINDINGS

The purpose of this study was to generate hypothetical propositions about the ways in which the elderly interpret their world in a variety of settings. Three hypothetical propositions were created which are:

1. Rare moments of rebelliousness bear witness to the quiescent rage of the old.
2. Patterns of interrelating make manifest the automatic surrealism of the meaningless worlds of the old.
3. The thought of personal death lies always just at the surface of the explicit.

The findings indicate that growing old for the subjects in this study is a multidimensional complexity of the aging process as one

TABLE 9   HYPOTHETICAL PROPOSITIONS DERIVED FROM CONCEPTUAL CATEGORIES WITH THEIR PROPERTIES

CONCEPTUAL CATEGORY	PROPERTIES	HYPOTHETICAL PROPOSITION
I. Quiescent Rage	Estranged from vital centers of the everyday world Patronizing dismissal of self reliance Changing patterns of living	Rare moments of rebelliousness bear witness to the quiescent rage dormant in the old
II. Automatic Surrealism	Incessant waiting Mixed messages Meaninglessness	Patterns of interrelating make manifest the automatic surrealism of the meaningless worlds of the old.
III. Reluctant Readiness to Die	Emerging sense of uselessness Growing awareness of abandonment by own body Changing perception of self as when becoming increasing burden to family and others	The thought of personal death lies always just at the surface of the explicit

journeys toward the inevitability of non-being. Consistent with this view, proximity to the inevitability of non-being emerged from all of the settings. In fact, the similarities across settings were so striking that the researcher was led to speculate whether there is a culture of the old that transcends setting. The inevitability of non-being was revealed in four themes:

1. *Pervading sense of surrender of one's self to the system.*

This sense of abandoning one's self surfaced in most of the domains. It was characterized by a spirit of "going along" in order to insure that one would be cared for when it became necessary. It surfaced in the emerging perception of self as eventually inevitably helpless.

2. *Curiosity about, and interest in, the topic of death.*

This theme was highly visible in many of the domains and was articulated in graphically explicit as well as more subtle ways. It was characterized by mixed feelings which were related to the realization that life was nearing the end.

3. *Growing acceptance of meaningless time.*

This theme surfaced in many of the domains. It was characterized by a shift from subtle anger to sadness to indifference and finally to a kind of suspended waiting. It was made manifest in docile acceptance of incessant waiting.

4. *Dreaded images of a nursing home as a place to wait for death.*

This was a major theme closely related to many of the domains. It was characterized by emphatic beliefs that a nursing home was a place to go until death came.

The hypothetical propositions emerged from these themes. They are clearly related to the theory of Man-Living-Health, as articulated in Chapter II of this work. The interrelationship of the theory and the hypothetical proposition follows.

1. *Rare moments of rebelliousness bear witness to the quiescent rage dormant in the old.*

These rare moments are languaged as one stretches the meaning moment to transcend the ambiguity of the paradoxes and live the valued ideals. The quiescent rage ignites the spark of rebellion as different meanings emerge in new awarenesses of concrete realities. These new awarenesses power the originating of different ways of cocreating a livable experience.

2. *Patterns of interrelating make manifest the automatic sur-realism of the meaningless worlds of the old.*

Automatic surrealism is the staged artificiality that affirms the illusion of pretense. It is a way of transcending the meaningless world which emerges from the confrontation with personal limitation. The connecting-separating rhythm is lived in the monotony of sameness as one participates in the pretense of engagement which structures the meaning of reality.

3. *The thought of personal death lies always just at the surface of the explicit.*

The tacit-explicit meaning of dying is lived in the evolving everyday awareness of the proximity of death. The shifting rhythm of the distant closeness image of personal non-being cocreates opportunities to live the paradoxical struggle to persist in living. Living is the everchanging journey in the creation of new memories. Out of the remembered past, the aged transform the present toward what is yet to be.

It is evident from these hypothetical propositions that Man as living unity generates unique realities in ongoing participation with the world over time. The correspondence between the hypothetical propositions and the theory of Man-Living-Health as articulated above gives evidence of support of the theory.

VIII

THE DESCRIPTIVE METHOD

The descriptive method as a mode of inquiry originated in the social sciences. It is a method which yields findings based upon conversations and observations. It is a human science method which focuses on discovering the meaning of an event in time. Man develops a definition of the world through the experience of life events. The descriptive method includes an elaboration of the context of the situation, as well as the retrospective happenings and prospective plans surrounding the life event. The description, as told through the interrelationship between the researcher and the subjects, reflects the unitary nature of Man and the connectedness of Man with the environment. When a researcher seeks to study Man-environment interaction as a unit, the descriptive method is one method of choice. This method generates hypotheses for further research and enhances theory.

There are two types of descriptive methods presented in this work, the case study and the exploratory study. The case study is an in-depth investigation of a social unit, leading to a complete organized picture of it (Isaac and Michael, 1981). The case study tells the story of life events and allows the investigator to study a phenomenon as it is being lived and as it changes over time. The exploratory study is an investigation of the meaning of a life event for a group of subjects who shared a particular event.

PURPOSE

The purpose of the descriptive method is to intensively investigate the background and environmental interactions of a given social unit. A social unit is an organized entity having common characteristics. It can be one person, a family, or a set of persons or families

(Isaac and Michael, 1981). The study encompasses a macroscopic moment in time or a microscopic moment in time. The nature of the moment depends on the phenomenon guiding the study and the question posed in the study.

The descriptive method, like other qualitative and quantitative methods, is a research approach encompassing five basic elements. These are 1. identifying the phenomenon; 2. structuring the study; 3. gathering the data; 4. analyzing the data; and 5. describing the findings.

IDENTIFYING THE PHENOMENON

In the descriptive method, the phenomenon is a general proposition which guides the organization of the entire study, evolving from a particular frame of reference and setting the context for complete implementation of the study. The frame of reference set forth in Chapter II of this book relates to the lived experience of health. The lived experience of health is defined as structuring meaning, cocreating rhythmical patterns and cotranscending with the possibles (Parse, 1981). For example, some phenomena from the frame of reference might be: 1. participating knowingly incarnates opportunities for one who is dying; and 2. a family separation cocreates a paradoxical mix of sadness and joy.

STRUCTURING THE STUDY

Structuring the study plan includes specifying a research question, developing a conceptual framework, identifying the objectives of the study, identifying a study sample, and protecting the rights of subjects.

The Research Question

Research questions might be posed such as, "What opportunities are created when one participates knowingly in one's own dying?" and "What are the patterns of joy-sadness associated with separating in a family?" These questions are congruent with the nursing perspective articulated in Chapter II of this text. They focus on seeking an understanding of the lived experience of health.

Conceptual Framework

The conceptual framework provides the rationale for the study. It describes the phenomenon from a particular paradigmatic perspective of nursing and, as such, guides the subsequent phases of the study. The conceptual framework is a creative synthesis invented by the researcher. It arises from disciplined persistence in coming to know and understand the phenomenon, and occurs while engaging in the rhythmical process of analyzing-synthesizing while in a contemplative mood.

The conceptual framework is a logical construction, derived from a knowledge base, and supported by congruent references. It contains propositions which flow logically through a complete explanation of the essences of the phenomenon.

The objectives of the study flow from the conceptual framework and specify the parameters of data gathering and analysis. An objective includes both a content and a process component. It identifies a single activity related to one element of the phenomenon. For example, two objectives might be: to describe the joy-sadness pattern in a family separation event; and to describe the opportunities created by one who participates knowingly in dying.

Study Sample

In the descriptive method, the sample is drawn from the population experiencing the phenomenon being studied. The sample is comprised of a social unit which may be an individual, family or group.

Protecting the Rights of Human Subjects

Subjects are invited to participate and are given an explanation of the study and of what their participation entails, including information about confidentiality, anonymity, and the option to withdraw from the study at any time.

DATA GATHERING

Data may be gathered through interview, observation, or questionnaire. Interview is a face-to-face encounter between researcher and subject in which the subject shares specific information related to the objectives of the study. Interview questions derived from the objectives are written clearly and succinctly. They are open ended and directed toward uncovering the meaning of the lived experience under study. For example, a question used in uncovering the meaning of the lived experience of retirement is "How has retirement changed the way you talk to each other?"

Observation is a direct or indirect method of witnessing an activity for the purpose of recording information related to the objectives of the study.

The questionnaire is a structured technique designed for the purpose of gathering information in an organized fashion. It is a tool, derived from the objectives of the study, which contains clearly stated self-explanatory interrogatory statements. The questions are carefully designed to elicit specific data consistent with the purpose of the study. The content of these three methods of data collection is derived from the objectives of the study, and the data are the actual interactions collected through these methods.

DATA ANALYSIS

Data analysis in the descriptive method begins with a careful examination of the subject-researcher interaction, which entails a search for major themes articulated by the subjects about the phenomenon. This occurs through analysis-synthesis. Analysis-synthesis is a process of separating the themes according to the major elements in the objectives, examining these elements, and constructing a unified description of the phenomenon as lived by the subjects. The major themes are transformed to a higher level of discourse in the move from the subjects' language to the language of the researcher.

In case studies, the themes in the language of the subjects are interrelated to form a coherent, integrated reconstruction of the unit of study, and then are synthesized and transformed into a hypothetical statement. The themes in the exploratory study are synthesized into hypothetical statements related to the objectives of the study.

The themes in exploratory studies are synthesized directly into hypothetical statements.

DESCRIBING THE FINDINGS

The findings of a study using the case method incorporate the integrated reconstruction of the unit of study and the synthesized hypothetical statements. In reporting the findings, the case (that is, the story) is presented. A case study follows in Chapter 9.

The findings of an exploratory study are the hypothetical statements. In reporting the findings, the generated hypotheses are set forth. An exploratory study follows in Chapter 10.

IX

The Experience of Retirement
A Case Study

Purpose

The purpose of this study is to describe the experience of retirement through an in-depth study of a social unit, the family. The rationale for choosing the case study is that this method is directed toward discovering the meaning of a life event as it is being lived over time.

Research Question

This investigation sought to answer the question, What are the health patterns associated with retiring?

Phenomenon

The phenomenon central to this study is the proposition that significant life events rhythmically cocreate reaching beyond. This means that life events viewed as critical are manifested in an ebb and flow which leads beyond the event to the not-yet. The critical element in an event is identified in the meaning given to the event by the individual. No event is critical in itself. The ebb and flow is a synchronous process which surfaces new meaning and thrusts one from the event to different possibles. The choice of retirement as a critical event surfaced as a result of a small scale study designed to be consistent with the assumption that health is cocreated in the Man-environment interchange. The findings of this small scale study revealed that:

1. Significant life events included retirement, death of a spouse, and marriage.

2. Caring patterns were revealed as sharing burdens and joys with others.

3. The importance of ordering each day included making specific plans.

CONCEPTUAL FRAMEWORK

The conceptual framework that served as a rationale for the study and explained the phenomenon was the theory of Man-Living-Health (Parse, 1981). Health is cocreated in the process of the Man-environment interchange. The lived experience of health is the way in which Man cocreates the living of valued priorities. Value priorities are lived with the options, important others, and dreams of everydayness. Concepts of greater specificity were derived from each principle through the process of logical mapping. Table 10 depicts the logical mapping of each principle.

Meanings are given in situations as one simultaneously lives the processes of interpretation, signification, and explication in the making of everyday choices. All life events for an individual have personal meanings that are assigned by the individual. The meaning given reflects values and cherished beliefs and are languaged in patterns of expression. Health is rooted in the significance, interpretation, and explication given to the choices associated with life events.

Relationships are the rhythmical Man-environment interchanges expressed through revealing-concealing, enabling-limiting, and connecting-separating. These are reflected in the presence and non-presence of important others. Relationships are related to the quality of disclosure in revealing-concealing, the directional movement in enabling-limiting, and the nearness of connecting-separating in the links with important others.

Cotranscendence is reaching beyond what is to what can be. Possibles point to the dreams that are not yet. Dreams are articulated in the imaging and languaging of the possibles as one invents ways to power in transforming toward that which is not yet.

TABLE 10   LOGICAL MAPPING OF PRINCIPLES OF MAN-LIVING-HEALTH*

PRINCIPLE I.   STRUCTURING MEANING MULTIDIMENSIONALLY IS COCREATING REALITY
THROUGH THE LANGUAGING OF VALUING AND IMAGING.

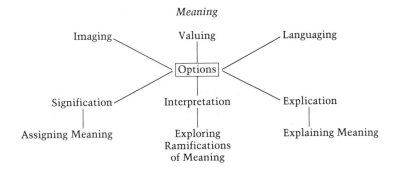

Meaning

Imaging   Valuing   Languaging

Options

Signification   Interpretation   Explication

Assigning Meaning   Exploring   Explaining Meaning
Ramifications
of Meaning

PRINCIPLE II.   COCREATING RHYTHMICAL PATTERNS OF RELATING IS LIVING THE PARA-
DOXICAL UNITY OF REVEALING-CONCEALING AND ENABLING-LIMITING
WHILE CONNECTING-SEPARATING.

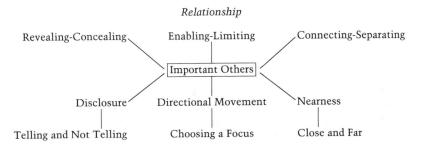

Relationship

Revealing-Concealing   Enabling-Limiting   Connecting-Separating

Important Others

Disclosure   Directional Movement   Nearness

Telling and Not Telling   Choosing a Focus   Close and Far

PRINCIPLE III.   COTRANSCENDING WITH THE POSSIBLES IS POWERING UNIQUE WAYS OF
ORIGINATING IN THE PROCESS OF TRANSFORMING.

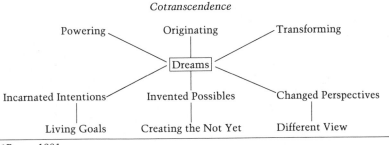

Cotranscendence

Powering   Originating   Transforming

Dreams

Incarnated Intentions   Invented Possibles   Changed Perspectives

Living Goals   Creating the Not Yet   Different View

*Parse, 1981

Objectives

The objectives for this study were:

1. To describe the unfolding health patterns related to signification, interpretation, and explication of the lived experience of retiring;

2. To describe the unfolding health patterns in relation to disclosure, directional movement, and nearness in the lived experience of retiring;

3. To describe the unfolding health patterns in relation to intentions, invented possibles and changed perspectives in the experience of retiring.

SAMPLE

The sample chosen as the social unit for this case study consists of a married couple who have experienced retirement. Each member of the couple retired at the same time and has been retired for the past two years. The couple have been married for 20 years and have lived in a rural community during their marriage.

PROTECTION OF SUBJECTS' RIGHTS

The couple was provided with an explanation of the study which included the time involved in their participation. They understood that the data would be tape recorded and used for a research study and that their identity would remain anonymous in the presentation of the study. The couple consented to participate.

DATA GATHERING

The data were gathered through personal unstructured interviews which were tape recorded. The guide questions were derived directly from the research objectives and they are as follows:

Meaning

1. *Signification—Assigned Meaning*
What did you think of retirement before you retired? Tell me what retirement means to you. What seems most important to you?

2. *Interpretation—Exploring Ramifications*
Talk to me about how you think and feel about these important matters related to retirement.

3. *Explication—Explaining Meaning*
How are these things important to you?

Relationships

4. *Disclosure—Telling and Not Telling*
How has retirement changed the way you talk to each other? Are you able to share issues with each other?

5. *Movement—Choosing a way to move*
How did you decide this way of sharing with each other was a change?

6. *Nearness—Close and Far*
Tell me about how retirement has changed your relationship with each other and with others who are important to you.

Transcendence

7. *Intentions—Living Goals*
What are your plans?

8. *Invented Possibles—Creating the not yet*
What are your dreams? How do you intend to make them come true?

9. *Changed Perspective—Different View*
What things do you see more clearly now? Since retirement what views of life have changed for you?

The complete transcript of the data appears in Appendix C.

DATA ANALYSIS

Data analysis began with careful examination of the researcher-subject interactions. These interactions were synthesized into the following reconstructed case.

The Case

Neither Mr. nor Mrs. E had a definite plan for retirement. For Mr. E, the outside world said to him, "don't retire," while his body was saying, "retire." For Mrs. E, a change in relationships in the work situation led to retirement. Both persons in the couple retired at about the same time and each had made his/her own decision to retire. Mr. E. chose to retire because of the increased hassle associated with his job and because pain in his leg was "getting to be too much." Mrs. E retired because her job situation changed and retirement was viewed as a relief from the burden and monotony associated with work. Retirement was a choice both had freely made and looked forward to. Most important to them was the relief of hassle, but both said they enjoyed their work and missed the relationships at work. Also important was more time together to enjoy life. They look forward to eating out, traveling, and spending more time together. They are free to come and go as they please. They attend reunions of groups they belonged to before retirement, go shopping, and visit friends and relatives. Along with having more time together, they do different things with each other than they did before retiring. They also said that it is good to be apart from each other once in a while to pursue their own interests. The sudden death of a young neighbor who was close to them was a recent, painful experience. This event has created a change for them, as they no longer have a close neighbor to depend on. Both said they have a better view of life since retirement. There are fewer worries, problems, and hassles. For twenty years, Mr. E had indigestion and abdominal pain which are no longer present. Mrs. E feels closer to her husband and finds that things go more smoothly. They now talk together more and about more important things, such as commonly experienced events and their observations of others. Both read more and find more time to enjoy personal activities like playing the organ and gardening. Boredom is transcended by walks and visits. They are planning to investigate senior citizen events and volunteer work, and Mrs. E wants to take organ lessons. There is more time to be in the present for Mr. E, and Mrs. E has more time to be concerned about the future since retirement.

Major themes emerged through a careful examination of the data. The raw data were also examined by another person to verify the themes. These themes were then sorted under each objective. The following themes are those that emerged from the data according to each objective.

Themes in the Language of the Subject

OBJECTIVE 1. To describe the unfolding health patterns related to signification, interpretation and explication of the lived experience of retirement.

Themes

    A. The outside world kept saying don't retire, yet body was saying retire.

    B. There was monotony and burden with work and retirement was a relief.

    C. Enjoyed some aspects of work yet other aspects were a hassle.

    D. Before retirement the rigorous time schedule created tiredness and little enjoyment; this was relieved after retirement.

    E. Both members of the family made their own decision to retire.

    F. Both members feel good about the freely chosen decision to retire since they both could still work if they choose to.

OBJECTIVE 2. To describe the unfolding health patterns in relation to disclosure, directional movement, and nearness in the lived experience of retiring.

Themes

    A. There is more time together with each other since retiring.

    B. They do different things together than they did before retirement.

    C. They have the freedom to come and go as they choose.

    D. They spend more time with relatives.

    E. They enjoy taking time to be apart and pursue their own interests.

OBJECTIVE 3. To describe the unfolding health patterns in relation to intentions, invented possibles and changed perspectives in the experience of retiring.

Themes

    A. They believe life is short and you only live one day at a time.

    B. Their observations of some others conflict with their own experience of retirement.

    C. Boredom is transcended by driving, walking, and visiting.

    D. Their view of life is much better since retirement.

    E. Their life is smoother.

F. They are grateful for what they have.

G. There is more time to be in the present.

H. They plan to increase their participation with others through volunteer work and senior citizen activities.

I. They are happy with the way they are, although she dreams of being closer to her family but does not want to move.

Themes in the Language of the Researcher

The themes under each objective in the language of the subject were transformed to a higher level of discourse in the language of the researcher. One theme was synthesized in relation to each objective.

OBJECTIVE 1.   To describe the unfolding health patterns related to signification, interpretation and explication of the lived experience of retiring.

Theme 1.

An emerging clarity toward being unencumbered surfaced through the paradoxical mist.

OBJECTIVE 2.   To describe the unfolding health patterns in relation to disclosure, directional movement, and nearness in the lived experience of retiring.

Theme 2.

A changing spatial-temporal rhythm created a more complex interconnectedness.

OBJECTIVE 3.   To describe the unfolding health patterns in relation to intentions, invented possibles, and changed perspectives in the lived experience of retiring.

Theme 3.

A shifting perspective expanded the view of what is possible.

In the process of analysis-synthesis with the objectives, reconstructed case, and themes, the researcher identified the following health patterns related to retirement.

1. A freely chosen decision,

2. A shift in the rhythm of the relationship,

3. A change in view of life.

These health patterns are related to man's negentropic unfolding in health.

DISCUSSION OF THE FINDINGS

The lived experience of retirement for this couple was a self-directed, freely chosen decision made in the context of hassle, rigid schedules, work pressures, and monotony. The couple was pleased and relieved with the decision to retire which allowed them more time together, as well as some time apart. They were talking more to each other and things were going smoothly. They intended to extend their relationships with others and viewed life as better since retiring. The following hypothesis flows from the case analysis-synthesis and reflects the meaning of retirement for the couple.

Retirement is a *freely chosen* experience which leads to a *shift in meaning and relationships* generating the *exploration of possibilities.*

The hypothesis is clearly related to the theory of Man-Living-Health (Parse, 1981). Man is an open being in continuous interchange with the environment, choosing and being accountable for, choices. Man is both enabled and limited by choices; that is, to choose retirement is to give up the life pattern of working and to take on the life pattern of retirement without knowing the outcome of the decision. The decision to retire is a personal choice and a confrontation with the being-wondering paradox. This being-wondering paradox for both persons in the couple was the struggle with what was present at the time for them, and what might be present with retirement. In the process of struggling with the decision, the outcome was sometimes clear and sometimes hazy. The couple were constantly called to be relieved of the burdensome schedule. Each took responsibility for making his and her own decision.

A shift in meaning and relationships is a coconstituted rhythm of the open Man-environment interchange. The ebb and flow of both meaning and relationships changed in the decision to retire. Health is man's becoming in the shifting rhythms cocreated as Man and environment interrelate (Parse, 1981). The cocreated shifting rhythms of the Man-environment interchange involves changing from what one is to what one struggles to become. The struggle to become is lived in the changing dimensions of space-time. The decision to retire shifted the meaning and relationship rhythms of the becoming Man-environment interchange.

Possibilities unfold in the Man-environment interchange. Unique possibilities emerge as Man integrates the unfamiliar with the familiar. As changes in personal meanings and relationships expand, the view of what is possible for Man grows in complexity. This is related to the assumption that health is unitary Man's negentropic unfolding (Parse, 1981).

The correspondence between the generated hypothesis and the theory of Man-Living-Health, offers support for the theory. This generated hypothesis offers the opportunity to further investigate the phenomenon using different methods.

X

THE MEANING OF
BEING EXPOSED TO TOXIC CHEMICALS
AN EXPLORATORY STUDY*

PURPOSE

The purpose of this descriptive study was to explore the meaning of the experience of living through an environmental toxic emergency. As each subject spoke of his feelings, thoughts, and perceptions concerning the exposure to toxic chemicals, the personal meaning of health surfaced.

The descriptive exploratory study was the method of choice because it focuses on the discovery of the meaning of experience through interview, which provides a first hand account of life events. The method offers an opportunity to discover common health patterns from a number of subjects who participated in the same event.

RESEARCH QUESTION

This investigation sought to answer the question: What is the meaning of being exposed to potential carcinogens for firefighters, eighteen months after the incident?

---

*Extrapolated from a research study completed by Carol Z. Weiner and reported here with permission.

PHENOMENON

The phenomenon central to this study is the proposition that health is languaging the powering of the enabling-limiting paradox. This means that one's way of being shows itself in the interhuman struggles of making choices which both enhance and restrict progress simultaneously. One's health is the way one lives interhuman struggles in life events.

CONCEPTUAL FRAMEWORK

Man languages the meaning of a particular lived experience through powering possibles. This study, which investigates the meaning of the lived experience of being exposed to potential carcinogens, is guided by the following phenomenon: Health is languaging the powering of the enabling-limiting paradox. This proposition, which emerges from the principles of the work, *Man-Living-Health: A Theory of Nursing* by Rosemarie Rizzo Parse, will provide the conceptual framework for this study. Parse (1981) identifies "unitary Man as one who coparticipates with the environment in creating and becoming, and who is whole, open, and free to choose ways of living health" (p. 7). She identifies health "as ongoing participation with the world . . . a unitary phenomenon that refers to Man's becoming through cocreating rhythmical patterns of relating in open energy interchange with the environment . . . unitary Man's health is a synthesis of values, a way of living" (p.39). Health, then, is the choice of how one will be as one lives in the world.

There are three major concepts in the proposition guiding this study: languaging, powering, and enabling-limiting.

Languaging is a process of expressing valued images. Merleau-Ponty (1974) writes that language is a transforming of a certain kind of silence into speech. "The spoken word is a gesture, and its meaning, a world" (p. 184). Parse (1981) states "When one person encounters another person, rhythmical patterns of relating unfold as words become sentences and are shared with a certain volume and a particular tempo with unique intonation, simultaneously with a certain gaze, gesture, touch, and posture" (p. 47-48). Other dimensions of languaging are the "rhythmical moments of silence, the choice of words and syntax, the intonation, the facial expressions, the gestures, the posture and that which is not said that constitute the symbolic expression which is characteristic of languaging as a concept of structuring meaning multidimensionally" (pp. 46-47).

The second concept guiding this study is powering. Powering is a process of Man-environment interchange recognized in the continuous affirming of self in light of the possibility of non-being. Tillich (1954) states that "power is the possibility of self-affirmation in spite of internal and external negation" (p. 40). Parse (1981), congruent with Tillich, says "being is continuously confronted with non-being. Non-being refers not only to dying but to the risk of losing one's self through being rejected, threatened, or not recognized in a manner consistent with expectations" (p. 57). Parse also states that "powering patterns unfold in Man-other interrelationships and show themselves through languaging" (p. 37). Tillich (1954) says, "Power is the drive for everything living to realize itself with intensity and extensity" (p. 36). He further states that "Life is tentative. Everybody and everything has chances and must take risks, because his and its power of being remain hidden if actual encounters do not reveal it" (p. 41). "How one lives powering," Parse says, "is reflected in one's patterns of relating with the world through the rhythm of pushing-resisting. Pushing-resisting is in every human encounter, creating tension and conflict that create the alternatives from which one can choose in reaching beyond" (p. 37). The choices one powers through pushing-resisting are related to affirming self over non-being.

The third concept in the proposition guiding this study is the enabling-limiting paradox. Parse (1981) states that the enabling-limiting paradox is a rhythmical pattern of Man-Living-Health. It shows that man in situation is simultaneously enabled and limited by choice. Man's choices are made at some risk. All outcomes are not fully known when choices are made. Sartre (1956) says that persons are free to make choices even though they do not necessarily have "the ability to obtain the ends chosen" (p. 459). Parse (1981) says, "Enabling-limiting is evident as Man chooses to be certain ways in situation. In this choosing Man enables self to move in one direction and limits movement in another" (p. 53). Man creates possibilities as choices are lived. "Man cannot be all possibilities at once and, in choosing, one is both enabled and limited" (Parse, 1981, p. 53). The choosings are options which carve out the not-yet.

These three major concepts then, languaging, powering, and enabling-limiting, discussed above reveal the meaning of the proposition, health is languaging the powering of the enabling-limiting paradox.

The major concepts are also the major descriptive elements of this study. Languaging is the firefighters' description of the silent disaster experience as determined by volume, tempo, intonation, word choice, silence, and syntax. Powering is the firefighters' view of self with the silent disaster situation, as determined by identification of statements of self-affirmation and self-negation. Enabling-limiting is the firefighters' view of the future as determined by identification of statements of choices related to the future.

OBJECTIVES

OBJECTIVE 1. To describe the languaging of exposure to potential carcinogens, as lived by firefighters, through speech, including volume, tempo, intonation, choice of words, silence, and syntax.

OBJECTIVE 2. To describe powering in relation to the exposure to potential carcinogens, as lived by firefighters, through the identification of themes as they surface in statements of self-affirmation and self-negation.

OBJECTIVE 3. To describe enabling-limiting in relation to the exposure to potential carcinogens by firefighters through identification of choices related to the future.

SAMPLE

The sample studied was comprised of seven volunteers of the total accessible population of the twenty-three firefighters who were exposed to polychlorinated byphenyls (PCBs), a potential carcinogen in humans, and proven carcinogen in test animals. The subjects, all male and married, ranging in age from 32 to 52, were exposed to these chemicals as they extinguished a fire in the basement of the state office building in a northeastern city with a population of 60,000.

PROTECTION OF SUBJECTS' RIGHTS

The details of the subjects' participation in the study were explained to them and each subject signed a consent form. All were aware of the provisions for confidentiality and anonymity and of the option to withdraw.

DATA GATHERING

An interview guide was used for investigating the meaning of this experience of being exposed for the firefighters. (See Appendix D1.)

The fire chief was contacted about the participation of the twenty-three firefighters exposed to potential carcinogens. He indicated that seven of the twenty-three volunteered to be subjects for the study. The informed consent form was signed by each subject and witnessed by another person. The interviews were done in a private area in each fire station. The meaning of the experience as it related to health emerged as the subjects spoke about their feelings, thoughts, and perceptions about the incident and its effect on their lives and the lives of their families. Each interview was tape recorded and later transcribed for analysis.

DATA ANALYSIS

Data were elicited from seven subjects. Each response from each subject on each question was analyzed and summarized. Then these responses were examined for patterns of languaging, themes related to powering, and statements related to choices for the future.

Statements related to powering, that is, self-affirmation and self-negation, surfaced in recurring themes. Enabling-limiting was shown in paraphrases or direct quotes dealing with choices relating to the future. Languaging was identified through speech, including volume, tempo, intonation, choice of words, silence, and syntax.

Presentation of Data

The data are presented in two parts; first, responses to the specific open-ended questions from the interview guide are shown by summarizing the essential points in paraphrases or direct quotes. (See Appendix D2.) Second, the data are presented according to the categories of this study: languaging, powering, and enabling-limiting. A general description of each subject's languaging is presented below. Languaging patterns are then shown in columns beside the statements which indicate the four themes that surfaced in analysis of the self-affirmation and self-negation statements as well as in columns beside the statements revealing the choices related to the future. (See Appendices D3 and D4.)

OBJECTIVE 1. To describe the languaging of the exposure to potential carcinogens as lived by firefighters, through speech, including volume, tempo, intonation, choice of words, silence, and syntax.

The following is a description of each subject as he languaged health.

SUBJECT 1 spoke in an even tempo. The volume of his voice was average and the pitch and tone were low throughout the interview. He sat relaxed at a table and maintained eye contact with the interviewer. At times, as the subject spoke, anger was reflected as the tempo of his voice became faster, the tone louder, and as each word was emphatically spoken. He used words like frustration and anger, his sentences were well structured, and there were few moments of silence.

SUBJECT 2 spoke calmly and reflectively with many periods of silence. As he spoke, he gazed out of the window, glancing occasionally at the interviewer. His voice was slow, the tone and volume low. As the interview progressed, the interviewer noted an increase in tempo and tone as words were being more emphatically spoken.

SUBJECT 3 was calm, and seemed uninterested in the interview. He spoke in a monotone, the volume and tone were low. He spoke as if he had no interest in the incident of the fire at the state office building. However, the choice of words indicate that he had similar concerns as the other subjects. There were frequent moments of silence but his sentences flowed with little hesitancy.

SUBJECT 4 was concerned at first about having the interview tape recorded. He did, however, consent to participate. He sat on the arm of the chair and, when invited to sit in the chair, refused. He was visibly tense, the muscles in his face twitched as he spoke. His voice was high-pitched, he spoke at a fast tempo, and he avoided eye contact with the interviewer. He repeated that he never thinks about the incident. The subject interrupted his own sentences frequently with different thoughts, and seemed to have difficulty continuing with ideas as he spoke.

SUBJECT 5 sat calmly as he spoke. The tone of his voice was high-pitched, he spoke in rapid sentences with many pauses. The choice of words clearly indicated the anxiety felt by this subject. He hesitated as he spoke, as if searching for words to complete sentences.

SUBJECT 6 spoke in an even tempo and low tone. As the interview progressed he spoke more quitely, but most of his speech was in a monotone and many sentences were not completed. He sat calmly and maintained eye contact with the interviewer. There were some moments of silence.

SUBJECT 7 spoke in a monotone. The tempo and tone of his voice were even and low, but when he began to speak of his anger the tone became lower and the tempo slower. His choice of words clearly indicated anger and his sentences were uninterrupted. The subject sat calmly and maintained eye contact with the interviewer.

OBJECTIVE 2.   To describe powering in relation to the exposure to potential carcinogens as lived by firefighters, through the identification of themes as they surface in statements of self-affirmation and self-negation.

For all seven subjects, health was experienced as each spoke of feelings, thoughts, and perceptions concerning the incident of the fire. Four themes related to powering (self-affirmation/self-negation) were identified. These themes are:

A.   Suspicious sense of impending danger,

B.   Disillusionment with the system,

C.   Explicit and implicit references to mortality,

D.   Distrust of experts.

These themes are aligned with languaging patterns in Appendix D3.

OBJECTIVE 3.   To describe enabling-limiting in relation to the exposure to potential carcinogens by firefighters, through identification of choices related to the future.

Statements related to the future made by the subjects were analyzed and synthesized. Three synthetic statements related to enabling-limiting representative of the overall view of the future for these subjects were identified according to Objective 3: These are:

A.   Continuing commitment to vocation of firefighting in light of known risks,

B.   Reluctant willingness to engage in similar situation,

C.   Choosing carefully among changing patterns in close relationships.

These statements are aligned with languaging patterns in Appendix D4.

DISCUSSION OF FINDINGS

The hypothesis generated from this study is that the lived experience of health in a silent disaster, for these subjects, is the confrontation with personal finitude intensified by a context of disillusionment with the system which mobilized closeness in personal relationships. The risk of confronting personal finitude showed itself as the subjects chose to remain as firefighters in light of the explicit knowledge about present dangers and future unknowns. While immersed in the present dangers which were intensified by distrust of the experts, the subjects seized the opportunity to re-examine relationships with close others and were moved to deepen them.

The hypothesis is clearly congruent with the proposition guiding this study which emerged from the principles of Man-Living-Health (Parse, 1981). The proposition that health is languaging the powering of the enabling-limiting paradox is connected to risk, personal finitude, and closeness.

Risk is shown in the struggles of the pushing-resisting rhythm in choosing alternatives which both enhance and restrict movement. The risk surfaces as one encounters personal finitude which is experienced in the choosing of being in the face of non-being. This choosing is living the enabling-limiting paradox which guides one to uncover hidden dimensions of interrelatedness. In uncovering the hidden dimensions, new meanings arise which power the possibility for richer relationships with close others.

The findings of this study give evidence of support for the theory of Man-Living-Health.

XI

CRITERIA FOR EVALUATION OF QUALITATIVE RESEARCH

E valuation of scholarly work is inherent in the evolution of all disciplines. It provides a consistent standard in the birthing of new knowledge and enhances the quality of the discipline.

Critical appraisal of research is essential for developing the science of nursing. It ensures a consistency through the application of standards of excellence. Critical appraisal is the judgment of value in light of particular standards of excellence. Judging involves the processes of interrogating and contrasting, used to systematically examine each component of the research study in light of a critique framework which specifies standards of excellence. The standards of excellence are definitive statements that set forth the essential elements in a research study. They guide evaluation of research studies and offer an overview of expectations which provide the impetus for refinement and bring to light the relative merit of a work in the development of nursing science.

Evaluation, in critical appraisal, has been a part of nursing's emergence as a science. The available critique frameworks in nursing are directed toward quantitative research studies. This is understandable in an era when most nursing research is quantitative in nature. With the emergence of the simultaneity paradigm and use of qualitative research methods, different criteria are required which reflect the different view of the paradigm and the methods. Criteria for evaluation, then, must reflect the basic assumptions of the research approach being used. There are two major research approaches defined in Chapter I of this text. The criteria in the critique framework set forth in this chapter are congruent with the qualitative approach, which is aligned with the simultaneity nursing paradigm. This critique framework evolved from a synthesis of Batey's (1977) analysis of the research process and Kaplan's (1964) norms of validation.

The critique framework includes standards and dimensions. The specific standards, Substance, Clarity and Integration, were created for the critique framework and aligned with the dimensions (Conceptual, Ethical, Methodological, and Interpretive) of the research process. A description of the standards follows:

SUBSTANCE

Substance reflects the soundness of ideas supported by evidence appropriate to the study. It includes the presentation of adequate details to support the major ideas under investigation. These ideas connect in a way that reflects correspondence to the existing knowledge base in nursing. There is evidence of appropriate movement of ideas up and down the levels of abstraction throughout the study. Major ideas are differentiated and thoroughly developed.

CLARITY

Clarity reflects distinct logical precision in presentation of ideas. It includes use of the right words in the correct grammatical structure. Major ideas are set forth in an organized, succinct way.

INTEGRATION

Integration reflects the flow of ideas in a coherent fashion. There are appropriate transitions between the major elements of the study. Integration includes a unified presentation which gives form to the study as a whole. Major ideas are structured logically to enhance development of the study.

The major dimensions of the research process delineate the process.

CONCEPTUAL DIMENSION

The conceptual dimension sets forth the phenomenon, research question, and frame of reference. It provides a guide for the structure and implementation of the study. Conceptualizations lead to expansion of the body of nursing knowledge through development of research studies that are derived from the works of nurse theorists.

ETHICAL DIMENSION

The ethical dimension includes the scientific merit of the research study and the protection of the rights of human subjects. The scientific merit of a study is judged on the basis of its overall value in the development of nursing science. The researcher has a responsibility to the scientific nursing community to ensure the integrity of the study from conceptualization through interpretation. The researcher must also protect the rights to self-determination of human subjects. Therefore, informed consent to participate in a study includes information about the details of the study, the risks and benefits of participating, the right to withdraw, protection from harm, and insurance of confidentiality.

METHODOLOGICAL DIMENSION

The methodological dimension includes the purpose, sample, data collection, and data analysis and is judged on the basis of the

TABLE 11   CRITIQUE FRAMEWORK

CRITERIA FOR CRITICAL APPRAISAL OF QUALITATIVE RESEARCH	
STANDARDS	DIMENSION
	Conceptual
Substance	How does the phenomenon relate to health?
	How is the phenomenon rooted in nursing knowledge?
	How does the frame of reference lead the reader to an understanding of the phenomenon?
	Does the frame of reference accurately reflect the referenced views?
Clarity	Is the phenomenon explicitly stated?
	Is the research question clearly stated?
	Is the research question an interrogative statement?
Integration	How does the research question flow from the phenomenon?
	How does the phenomenon and research question flow from the frame of reference?
	How is the frame of reference logically constructed?

(continued)

TABLE 11 *Continued*

CRITERIA FOR CRITICAL APPRAISAL OF QUALITATIVE RESEARCH

STANDARDS	DIMENSION
	Ethical
Substance	How does the study contribute to the scientific body of knowledge?
	How are the subjects' rights protected?
Clarity	Is the significance for nursing clearly stated?
	Is it clear how informed consent will be obtained?
Integration	Does the researcher stay true to the data?
	Methodological
Substance	How was the sample adequate with respect to the particular method?
	How is the data gathering process appropriate for the particular method?
	How does the researcher show the conceptual shifts in levels of abstraction?
	How do the abstract statements evolve from the raw data?
Clarity	Is the purpose of the method made clear by the researcher?
	Is the sampling process described clearly?
	Is the data collection method stated clearly?
	Is the process for data analysis made explicit?
	Are the findings of the study made explicit?
Integration	Are the basic principles of the method incorporated throughout the study?
	Is the data analysis process appropriate for the particular method?
	Interpretive
Substance	To what extent are the findings interpreted in light of the conceptualization of the study?
	How do the interpretive statements correspond with the findings?
	How do the interpretations reflect heuristic conceptualizations?
Clarity	Are the findings clearly interpreted in light of theory, research, and practice?
Integration	Does the interpretation take into consideration all of the other phases of the research process?

adequacy of the data to answer the research question. The adequacy of the data reflects the appropriateness of the method for studying the phenomenon. Correspondence of the method to the conceptualization is essential.

INTERPRETIVE DIMENSION

The interpretive dimension shows the findings in light of their pragmatic implications for theory development, research, and practice. The interpretation integrates coherently the findings of the study with the conceptualization. The interpretation also reflects heuristic conceptualizations.

Questions to be used in the critical appraisal of qualitative research studies follow in Table 11. The questions in the critique framework were generated in light of Batey's (1977) analysis and Kaplan's (1964) norms. This critique framework may be used in the systematic interrogation of qualitative nursing research studies. The vigilant and persistent interrogation of research according to standards will continue to build the body of knowledge in the discipline of nursing.

XII

THE LIVED EXPERIENCE OF REACHING OUT
A PHENOMENOLOGICAL INVESTIGATION*

PURPOSE

The purpose of this study is to investigate the phenomenon of *reaching out* as a lived experience. In this investigation, the structure of meaning of *reaching out* will be uncovered and, in this sense, will expand the understanding of this phenomenon. This study sought to answer the question: What is the structural definition of the lived experience of *reaching out*?

This study is significant to nursing in that it will explore a human experience related to health and thus will expand the body of nursing knowledge. The phenomenon will be explored in light of the researcher's perspective. The lived experience of *reaching out* to another evolves within Man to Man interrelationships.

RESEARCHER'S PERSPECTIVE

The researcher's perspective surfaced in a health crisis situation between the researcher and her mother. The researcher experienced *reaching out* as wanting to help her mother by lending strength and support through a difficult situation.

---

*Extrapolated from a research study completed by Nancy J. Andre and reported here with permission.

Reaching out, for the researcher, is powering the revealing-concealing of imaging (Parse, 1981). The essences of powering revealing-concealing and of imaging emerge in *reaching out*. Powering revealing-concealing is a way of investing one's energy to reach out to another in an interrelationship. In powering the revealing-concealing of *reaching out*, one chooses a way of interrelating with others. This way of interrelating is manifested in one's simultaneous revealing and concealing of self to others (Parse, 1981).

In *reaching out* one powers revealing-concealing in the way that discloses one's desire to extend to another. At the same time one conceals particular aspects of self. As one extends to another, a dynamic mutual coming together takes place. This extending can be described as a connecting or joining of one person with another. Kempler's (1974) idea of separating and unifying speaks of Man's endless search for relatedness to another. Kempler (1974) explains that separation and differentiation always lead to a union. In addition, unifying leads to separatedness and differentiation. This rhythmical process of separating and unifying is the happening (Kempler, 1974).

The rhythmical pattern of relatedness in *reaching out* can be described as a simultaneous uniting and separating of one with another. Mayeroff (1971) describes the essence of this rhythmical interrelationship in his discussion of caring. One experiences the other as an extension of oneself simultaneously as one experiences the other as separate from oneself, as having individual identity. One feels the other to be a part of oneself, yet recognizes the value and worth of the unique other in the other's own right.

Powering revealing-concealing involves risk. When one chooses to extend to another in *reaching out*, one accepts the risk inherent in one's choice. The choosing to come together in *reaching out* means that one risks a happening between oneself and another (Kempler, 1974). One risks not only the happening itself but all the consequences that may emerge from it. Mayeroff (1971) speaks of the risk in an interrelationship when he discusses trust. "Trusting the other is to let go; it includes an element of risk and a leap into the unknown, both of which take courage." As one moves to reach out to another, one reveals one's valuing of joining with another in an interrelationship. Simultaneously one conceals other values as one pushes to put forward one's desire to extend to another. This revealing and concealing of values involves risking one's being in the interrelationship. One risks possible rejection by another whose value system may be quite different from one's own (Parse, 1981).

Powering revealing-concealing is structured in the patterns and rhythms of *reaching out* with the other in a situation. One's chosen way of powering revealing-concealing in a situation takes on a particular pattern (Parse, 1981). In *reaching out* to another one chooses an intersubjective coming together. The *reaching out* leads to a sharing of one's being with the other in a partnership. The other is seen as a subject, a companion in the world. Viewing the other as an objective to be observed is a withdrawal of self and therefore not *reaching out*. Only when the other is a subject can one's wholeness of being be revealed to the other as an extension or reaching. Luijpen (1960) supports this concept of intersubjectivity in his discussion of persons as subjects and objects. In a later work (1964) he elaborates upon the very special way of one's presence to the other in his discussion of subjectivity and objectivity.

In powering the revealing-concealing of *reaching out*, one accepts the other as the other is and does not impose values. One regards the other as a unique person who has individual value and worth. Buber (1965) describes this process of unfolding to the other as a process of becoming, whereby one is guided by the other toward one's possibilities. Mayeroff (1971) describes caring as helping the other to grow. One experiences the other as having possibilities and the need to grow. One has a desire to unite with another so that one may enable the other's growth. This relationship is not one of dominance or dependence (Mayeroff, 1971). Instead, *reaching out* is a mutual nurturing of possibilities. The interrelationship is grounded in a mutual trust which enables the nurturing of possibilities to unfold. One enables the other's growth by not imposing one's own direction on the growth. One recognizes and respects the other's pattern of growth and in so doing guides one's own negentropic unfolding.

As one powers revealing-concealing in *reaching out*, one strives to be authentic in one's interrelationship with another. One does not pretend to be what one is not. One demonstrates openness in speaking what one feels and invites the other to share this genuine happening. This authenticity is supported by Buber (1965) when he speaks of coming together in an interrelationship as the "Between." He discusses the sphere of the interhuman and elaborates upon the duality of being and seeming. Buber (1965) explains that being leads to a genuine interhuman life while seeming leads to a life of false perspective.

The powering of revealing-concealing in *reaching out* emerges through one's imaging. One's creating of reality guides the direction of the interrelationship and gives it meaning. The desire to reach out to others has significance because one's experiences of *reaching out* have been structured into an interrelationship. One both tacitly and explicitly has meaningful knowledge about one's experiences of *reaching out* to others (Parse, 1981). This knowledge evolves and becomes more complex as one continues to reach out to others on a daily basis. One's reality, or worldview, is the foundation upon which the interrelationship builds. As one reveals and conceals one's imaged beliefs and values in *reaching out*, one continues to carve out one's meaningful cocreated reality (Parse, 1981).

METHOD

The method of study evolved from Giorgi's (1979) description of phenomenological analysis. This entails a written description of a lived experience by the subject, which is then interrogated by the researcher to uncover the meaning of the phenomenon.

SAMPLE

The sample for this research investigation consisted of two women, both of whom were between the ages of fifty and fifty-five. Subject Number One described a situation in which she illuminated the interrelationship with another person who wanted to learn to paint but thought it too difficult a task. Subject Number Two described a situation in which she illuminated her changing interrelationship with her husband. The sample size was limited to these two subjects for the purpose of this study.

Instructions to the Subjects

The subjects were initially contacted by the researcher. During the first contact, the researcher explained the purpose of the study and asked the subjects about their interest and willingness to participate. After giving verbal consent to participate in the study, the subjects were provided with written instructions that included the following:

> Describe a situation in which you experienced a mutual *reaching out* to another. Your description should include all your thoughts, feelings, and perceptions about the situation.

In addition, the subjects were asked to sign a document of informed consent in which they were assured that their rights of anonymity and confidentiality would be protected. The subjects were requested to complete their descriptions within one week. The researcher advised the subjects that they would be contacted at a later date for an elaboration of their descriptions. The subjects were informed that these elaborations would be tape recorded and transcribed by the researcher, and that the tapes would subsequently be destroyed.

DATA COLLECTION

The initial written descriptions obtained from the subjects were reviewed by the researcher in order to determine the areas where further elaboration was needed. Each subject's original description and elaborated description were combined.

RESULTS

The analysis of the data used the principles originally outlined by Spiegelberg (1976). Spiegelberg has described the process of investigating a particular phenomenon as including intuiting, analyzing, and describing. The phenomenological process of data analysis involves dwelling with the data, enabling the meanings to emerge while holding to the things themselves (Spiegelberg, 1976). Giorgi (1979) discusses this process and the following description of the analysis reflects his ideas.

Both descriptions were dwelled with and divided into naturally occurring units called scenes, which delineated the shifts in meanings within the descriptions. The themes or essences of the scene were described in the language of the subject. The researcher then dwelled with each theme in order to identify the focal meaning of each. The focal meanings were stated in the language of the researcher. To illustrate the researcher's conceptual shifts from raw data to focal meaning, examples of a scene, theme, and focal meaning for each subject follow:

Subject Number One

Scene

I said, "Well, B., why don't you take some painting lessons? Better still, I will take you to class with me. It just so happens that a new class is beginning next week." At first she said, "No, I may not be able to understand all the directions. Sometimes my English fails me and it is hard for me to explain," (She does have a kind of inferiority complex. She can't say R's and L's. The Japanese just do not have R's and L's. Many times if she can't understand something she will say, "How is that?" or "What is that?" She was afraid that in that class she would not understand and somebody would make little of that situation. I said, "No, no, nobody would do that. And if you have any trouble, I will help you." She said, "It is not even just that I would make the mistake, but maybe I won't understand if the instructor says to do such and such." I said, "Don't worry. If you can't understand that then I'll interpret for you. You can tell me what you think that means then I'll interpret that for you and we'll get that squared away.")

Theme

The subject offered to take her friend to painting class with her the next week. Her friend was negative toward her offer at first because she believed she would have some difficulty in understanding the directions given in class. She felt that her English was sometimes inadequate. The subject believed that her friend had an inferiority complex which was due to her difficulty with English. The subject felt that her friend feared being belittled in class and she reassured her that nobody would do that. The subject reassured her friend that she would help her through any difficulty she might have in class. She offered to interpret for her.

Focal Meaning

The subject experiences a desire to impose her values on the other in order to control the situation.

Subject Number Two

Scene

On January 17 and 18 we visited two attorneys both of whom stated for him not to separate, but he thought this was best as I took his self-esteem away from him and the children lost their father's image. He said he needed a thawing out period, to have his freedom and not be checked upon. A mutual separation was written out January 18, thereby leaving the house for six months or less and leaving the house in my name until such time that he arrived back with us. He left the premises on January 19. Much to my sorrow, in spite of it all, I can't live with him nor can I live without him. Through all these years am I confusing love with loneliness, always giving myself and not being recognized? (I think my husband appreciates me one hundred percent insofar as the home. He always said I was a perfectionist in the home. I was a perfectionist with the children. I feel that he didn't recognize me in the sense that he was always doing his own things, running out, running out—selfish in a respect. Not recognizing me as the other partner. We never went out together much in our last fifteen years as opposed to the first fifteen years. The last fifteen years our life style changed. So that somewhere along the line he more or less pushed on alone. He went on his own. In that respect I feel that I wasn't recognized. But I think he recognized me one hundred percent as being the wife and mother, in that respect, domesticated, or otherwise.)

The first week of separation he phoned. The purpose of the separation was to be totally away from each other, but I was glad to hear his voice and I knew in my heart by the sound of his voice that he missed me (or my Cinderella image). (I felt like we were together again. Even though it was a phone call, I felt like we were together again. He was *reaching out* for me and I was *reaching out* for him. And in spite of the separation I really feel that he wanted the separation to get himself cleared.) He's never brought up a legal paper with me so he is not really being fair to me. He is not even recognizing me as his wife because he is not putting his cards on the table and saying to me I did this or I did that. I feel in my heart why didn't he come to me? In fact, I even said to him I'll go to the attorney's office with you. I didn't care what it was or what he did. I feel I wanted to go with him. But he said, "I got myself into it and I'll get myself out of it." So that I'm still left out.

Theme

The subject's husband felt that a separation was necessary. A mutual separation was written out on January 18 and implemented on January 19. Much to the subject's sorrow, she cannot live with him, nor can she live without him. The subject feels that her husband did not recognize her in their marriage in that he did not see her as the other partner. During the first week of separation the subject received a telephone call from her husband. She was glad to hear his voice and she believed that her husband's voice reflected that he missed her also. The subject felt like they were together again *reaching out* to one another.

Focal Meaning

The subject acquiesces to the separation initiated by her husband; however, she soon afterward experiences a desire to be close to her husband again.

The focal meanings of each description were then synthesized into two situated structural descriptions. The situated structural descriptions detail the meaning of lived experience of *reaching out* for each subject in the situation. Both situated structural descriptions were then synthesized into one general structural description which represented the general structural meaning of the phenomenon of *reaching out* to another.

The focal meanings, situated structural descriptions, and the general structural description for both subjects will be presented here.

The scenes and themes are omitted in presentation of a qualitative study.

Subject Number One

For subject number one, nine themes emerged, which led to nine focal meanings:

Focal Meaning 1

For the subject *reaching out* is experienced in a friendly relationship with another in which selflessness is highly valued.

Focal Meaning 2

The subject is uplifted by the other's sense of awe which emerged from her prizing paintings through appreciation of the particulars.

Focal Meaning 3

The subject experiences a desire to impose her values on the other in order to control the situation.

Focal Meaning 4

The subject justifies taking over the situation and her desire to control the other.

Focal Meaning 5

The subject experiences confirmation as the other accepts her views with delight.

Focal Meaning 6

The subject experiences the other as choosing what she (subject) perceives to be a very difficult project, yet the subject justifies and affirms the other's choice.

Focal Meaning 7

The subject experiences jubilation in the knowledge that the other has reached a pinnacle.

Focal Meaning 8

The subject experienced utmost joy in having unveiled a source of enrichment for the life of another.

Focal Meaning 9

The subject bursts with a sense of fulfillment which she experienced as a euphoric elevation.

Subject Number One: Situated Structural Description

The focal meanings were synthesized into the situated structural descriptions. For this subject, the experience of *reaching out* to another emerged in a friendly relationship with another in which selflessness was highly valued. The subject described her friend as being very warm and sincere.

The subject had been doing oil painting as a hobby when one day her friend was visiting and admired some of her paintings. The friend expressed a desire to be able to paint as the subject did. The subject felt uplifted by the other's sense of awe which emerged from her prizing the paintings through appreciation of particulars.

The subject suggested to her friend that she could take her to painting classes with her as a new class was beginning. The friend initially declined the subject's offer and revealed her reason for declining. The subject persisted in her attempts to persuade her friend to take the painting lessons with her. The subject experienced a desire to impose her values on the other in order to control the situation.

The subject justified taking over the situation and her desire to control the other by stating that if she had been in her friend's place she would have wanted a friend to intervene as she had. The subject's friend eventually accepted her offer to accompany her to the painting classes. The subject experienced confirmation as the other accepted her views with delight.

On the first evening of the painting class the subject experienced her friend as choosing what she (subject) perceived to be a very difficult project, yet the subject justified and affirmed the other's choice. The other completed the difficult project with an intense sense of accomplishment. The subject felt a sense of jubilation in the knowledge that the other had reached a pinnacle.

The height of this experience for the subject emerged in her realization that she had unveiled a source of enrichment for the life of another. The subject experienced utmost joy in this knowledge. The subject was bursting with a sense of fulfillment which she experienced as a euphoric elevation.

Subject Number Two

For subject number two, four themes emerged from the description. The four themes led to four focal meanings:

Focal Meaning 1

For the subject the experience of *reaching out* is rooted in a longstanding marital connectedness in which she experiences a mixture of frustration with her husband's discontent and accomplishment for her high degree of commitment and personal sacrifice.

Focal Meaning 2

The subject experiences a feeling of betrayal at the extensive and obvious rejection by her husband which she attempted to justify and seek help for as the relationship became disconnected.

Focal Meaning 3

The subject acquiesces to the separation initiated by her husband, however, she soon afterward experiences a desire to be close to her husband again.

Focal Meaning 4

The subject experiences being torn as she and her husband reach out in different ways. She desires resuming connections yet is uncertain about her forgiveness of him.

Subject Number Two: Situated Structural Description

The focal meanings were synthesized into a situated structural description. For this subject, the experience of *reaching out* to another was rooted in a longstanding marital connectedness in which she experienced a mixture of frustration with her husband's discontent and accomplishment for her high degree of commitment and personal sacrifice. The subject believed that her relationship with her husband was no longer the happy one they enjoyed in the earlier years of their marriage. The subject noticed that her husband developed a pattern of consistently lying to her. She experienced a feeling of betrayal at the extensive and obvious rejection by her husband which she attempted to justify and seek help for as the relationship became disconnected. The subject's husband finally initiated separation proceedings. The subject acquiesced to the separation; however, she soon afterward experienced a desire to be close to her husband again.

Shortly after the separation the subject received a telephone call from her husband. As they talked together she recognized that they both expressed that they missed one another. The subject experienced being torn as she and her husband reached out in different ways. She desired resuming connections with her husband, yet she was uncertain about her ability to forgive him.

General Structural Description

A synthesis of the two situational structural descriptions led to the general structural description which explicated the meaning of *reaching out*. It is as follows:

> The experience of *reaching out* to another emerges in an interrelationship where one views self as committed to the welfare of another in a selfless way. One's commitment to another is lived in one's desire to make personal sacrifices in order to enrich the life of another.

Reaching out to another person involves the process of pushing-resisting. The energy of the pushing-resisting process is directed toward moving beyond the structure of the relationship. The connectedness of one with the other in the relationship shows disruption in the form of rejection of one by the other. This rejection or resisting is only temporary as one quickly moves to push the other again. This process demonstrates one's significant investment of energy to ensure the growth of the interrelationship.

The envisioned relationship in *reaching out* confirms an acceptance of self by the other. The knowledge that one is accepted by the other is essential to the growth of the interrelationship. This confirmation renews energies and serves as a process of revitalization.

DISCUSSION

The essential ideas that emerge from the general description of *reaching out* are as follows:

1. The experience of *reaching out* emerges in an interrelationship where one views self as committed to the welfare of another in a selfless way;

2. *Reaching out* involves the process of pushing-resisting in order to ensure the growth of the interrelationship;

3. One invests a significant amount of energy in the pushing-resisting process; and

4. The envisioned relationship in *reaching out* confirms an acceptance of self by the other which leads to a renewal of energies and serves as a process of revitalization.

The experience of *reaching out* emerges in an interrelationship where one views self as committed to the welfare of another in a selfless way. Each subject demonstrated a desire to make personal sacrifices in order to enrich the life of another. Mayeroff (1971) describes caring as helping the other to grow. Buber (1965) describes becoming as the process whereby one is guided by the other toward one's possibilities. Inherent in the idea of helping the other to grow toward possibilities is the concept of selflessness. As one nurtures the other's possibilities, one focuses one's energies on the other, rather than the self.

Reaching out involves the process of pushing-resisting in order to ensure the growth of the interrelationship (Parse, 1981). Each subject lived this pushing-resisting process in different ways. For the first subject, pushing-resisting was lived in her invitation to her friend to accompany her to painting classes and her friend's subsequent declination. The second subject lived pushing-resisting as she experienced a mixture of frustration with her husband's discontent and rejection, and accomplishment for her high degree of commitment to her marital responsibilities.

Kempler's (1974) idea of separating and unifying speaks of Man's endless search for relatedness to another. *Reaching out* involves a rhythmical pattern of relatedness that can be described as a simultaneous uniting and separating of one with the other. The process of simultaneous pushing-resisting in *reaching out* reveals a rhythmical pattern quite similar to separating and unifying (Parse, 1981).

One invests a significant amount of energy in the pushing-resisting process to enhance growth in a relationship. Both subjects made significant personal sacrifices for the welfare of the other. The degree to which each subject demonstrated a selfless commitment to the other signifies the energy that each put forth in the interrelationship. When the interrelationship showed disruption, each subject struggled through exerting individual efforts. Each subject centered energies upon the pushing-resisting process at hand.

One's investment of energy in the pushing-resisting process is related to the risk involved in the process of revealing-concealing (Parse, 1981). In the experience of *reaching out* one chooses to join with another in an interrelationship. As one makes the choice to reach out to another, one accepts the risk that is inherent in the choice. Mayeroff (1971) states that trusting the other includes an element of risk. He further states that risk requires courage. As one risks rejection in the process of pushing-resisting, one lives one's courage. One continuously invests significant amounts of energy in this process as one persists in risking in the interrelationship.

The envisioned relationship in *reaching out* confirms an acceptance of self by the other which leads to a renewal of energies and serves as a process of revitalization. Each subject experienced confirmation as the other demonstrated acceptance of the subject as a unique person. This acceptance of one's self by the other is a way of sharing one's being with another. Luijpen's (1969) discussion of intersubjectivity emphasizes the essentiality of subject-subject interactions in an authentic interrelationship.

The results which emerged from this study represent an approach toward expanding the nursing theory: Man-Living-Health (Parse, 1981). One principle, "Cocreating rhythmical patterns of relating is living the paradoxical unity of revealing-concealing and enabling-limiting while connecting-separating," is related to *reaching out* in that the rhythm of revealing-concealing is clearly a movement in engaging the other that discloses a part of self, as Subject One did for her friend and as Subject Two did for her husband. In disclosing a part of self one also conceals a part, yet risks being known and rejected (Parse, 1981). The principle, "Structuring meaning multidimensionally is cocreating reality through the languaging of valuing and imaging," is related to *reaching out* as a lived experience in that the envisioned relationship confirms an acceptance of self by the other and leads to a sense of renewal. Imaging how the relationship could be is the meaning given to the unselfish commitment to another. The principle, "Cotranscending with the possibles is powering unique ways of originating in the process of transforming," relates to the structural description of *reaching out* derived from this study in that the powering relationship is the interhuman pushing-resisting that thrusts one toward revitalization. This surfaces from the investment of energy in a relationship, and is directed toward growth. In this study, *reaching out* was found to involve the process of pushing-resisting in sustaining and nourishing the interrelationships over time.

IMPLICATIONS

The results of this study suggest that the experience of *reaching out* has implications for nursing practice through the development of the nursing theory: Man-Living-Health. The nurse has unique opportunities to identify family patterns of interrelating. *Reaching out* is one pattern of living Man/Man interrelationships that the nurse may illuminate with families. In light of these patterns, the nurse and family mobilize the implementation of strategies for change within the family's belief system. Strategies are used to guide change through illuminating, synchronizing and mobilizing energies.

The researcher suggests that future studies undertaken to investigate the phenomenon of *reaching out* include a larger sample for data analysis. Expanding the sample beyond the two subjects may enable new essences of *reaching out* to emerge. The sample could be expanded to include subjects of varying ages as well as both genders.

Further study of the phenomenon of *reaching out* might include an investigation of the ways one makes commitments to the welfare of another in a selfless way. Future studies would provide additional insight into the meaning of commitment in *reaching out*. For instance, one might ask subjects to:

Describe a situation in which you felt committed to another.

Describe a situation in which you felt committed to a thing or a project.

These descriptions could expand the meaning of the Man/Man and Man/environment interrelationships by exploring how Man commits self to people, things or projects.

XIII

ANDRE'S PHENOMENOLOGICAL INVESTIGATION OF REACHING OUT A CRITICAL APPRAISAL*

The critique is a powerful tool for dialogue within a scientific community. Critiques offer nurse scientists the opportunities to refine and appraise relationships between research and theory development through systematic evaluation of particular research studies and connections with specific nursing science frameworks. Furthermore, nursing as a professional discipline requires scholarly evaluation of research to promote prudent application of research findings in nursing practice.

The evaluation process is guided by predetermined standards of excellence identifying specific criteria against which the research work is judged. These criteria correspond to a specific research approach so that qualitative nursing studies are critiqued utilizing qualitative criteria that delineate standards within the broad dimensions of the conceptual, ethical, methodological and interpretative realms.

In this chapter, Andre's qualitative research study, *A Phenomenological Investigation of* [the lived experience of] *Reaching Out*, will be critiqued using Parse, Coyne, and Smith's criteria for evaluation of qualitative research. Each dimension will be evaluated in relation to the standards of substance, clarity, and integration, so that the work as a whole is judged according to the way theoretical and

---

*By Sharon J. Magan and Marlaine C. Smith.

empirical evidence is illuminated and incorporated within the research study and within nursing science.

CONCEPTUAL DIMENSION

The first research dimension involves the conceptual underpinnings of the phenomenon under study and its relationship to theory within the discipline of nursing. The phenomenon of *reaching out* is related to the way health is experienced within the complex interface of Man–Man relationships. *Reaching out* explores a pattern of interrelating with others.

Andre grounds the phenomenon of *reaching out* in nursing knowledge by using Parse's (1981) theory of Man-Living-Health in describing her frame of reference for the phenomenon. She essentially combines all three of Parse's principles by relating *reaching out* to the way one structures reality through imaging (Principle 1), to the rhythmical pattern of revealing-concealing (Principle 2), and to the transforming energy of powering (Principle 3). While the overall frame of reference refers to a major nurse theorist (Parse), Andre develops her perspective of the phenomenon of *reaching out* by detailing the views of other theorists who are consistent with Parse's perspective. The consistency between the concepts discussed confirms a theoretically accurate view of the phenomenon and leads the reader to a view of the researcher's perspective before a consideration of the research findings. That only one nurse theorist is cited by Andre can be understood when considering the relative newness of the simultaneity nursing paradigm and the subsequent paucity of research using this approach.

Andre's conceptual treatment of the phenomenon of *reaching out* is derived from concrete personal experience that illuminates *reaching out* as a distinct phenomenon that can be recognized in human patterns of interrelating. The theoretical support for her frame of reference is developed from scholarly sources. The research question is clearly stated in an interrogative form which flows from the identified phenomenon to be studied.

Andre's development of the frame of reference is sometimes obscure, in that the integration of the developed perspective does not occur until the end of the researcher's perspective. An introduction that incorporates the meaning of the essences of imaging, powering, and revealing-concealing would unite the essences as a whole with the phenomenon under study. Since the researcher's perspective has been clearly influenced by Parse's theory, a more explicit articulation of the concepts used from Parse would be helpful to the reader.

ETHICAL DIMENSION

The ethical dimension involves the subject's rights in participating in a scientific enterprise. The standard of substance in this dimension requires the researcher to substantiate the study's potential for contributing to nursing science so that the study is worthy of investigation and subject participation.

Andre described the significance of the study in terms of generating hypotheses related to health, as well as describing health through a detailed, empirically validated understanding of the lived experience of *reaching out*. The lack of generated hypotheses emerging from the research findings is a weakness in Andre's study.

Andre furnished specific guidelines for protecting the rights of subjects. She specified how the subjects were selected and approached and how informed written consent was obtained. She made explicit assurances to the subjects regarding anonymity and confidentiality.

The researcher's ethical responsibility extends into data analysis as the researcher proceeds to integrate focal meanings and derive structural descriptions of the phenomenon that accurately reflect the data directly provided by the subject's description. The examples provided illustrate the researcher's treatment of the data. Based on these examples, the reader can ascertain congruence between the subjects' descriptions and the focal meanings.

METHODOLOGICAL DIMENSION

The critique of the methodological dimension of Andre's study invites reflection on her application of the rigorous systematic phenomenological method. Andre assists the reader by articulating Spiegelberg's general essences.

Andre was clear in her description of the procedures and methods followed. She articulates the purpose of the phenomenological method. The sampling process was clearly described, as were specific details of the data collection process. Andre includes two subjects in the study. Although this number does fall within an acceptable range of a sample, Andre's study might be strengthened by analyzing more varied descriptions of the phenomenon. Andre suggests this in her implications for future research. The data collection procedure was appropriate. The use of the elaboration of the original written descriptions was a necessary adjunct to a richer understanding of the subjects' experiences. The steps of the data analysis procedure are clearly delineated and are appropriate.

Andre developed a question that asked the subject to describe an experience of mutually *reaching out*. While the mutual nature of *reaching out* is implicit in patterns of interrelating described in the researcher's perspective, it was not explicitly addressed. However, as a beginning investigation, it was perhaps retrospectively more valuable to ask subjects to focus on *reaching out* from a "mutual" approach. In this way the researcher was able to tap two different yet integrated perspectives of *reaching out*.

It is critical for the researcher to move logically from the concrete specific to the abstract realms as raw data meld into situated structural descriptions and finally into the general structural description of the phenomenon. The reader can readily ascertain the congruence between the scenes, themes, focal meanings, and respective situated structural descriptions. However, Andre's increasingly abstract descriptions of the phenomenon in the general structural description reveal some departures from the data and inconsistent progression into the abstract realms. For example, the appearance of pushing-resisting is difficult to relate to the focal meanings for Subject Number Two. Neither the subject's original frustration, betrayal, acquiescence to the separation, or desire for continuing connection represents a true sense of the semantic meaning of pushing-resisting. There is a weak association between the abstraction of pushing-resisting and the condition of participating in temporary disruptions or rejection in both subjects' relationships. The general structural description could be improved by both a more logical progression involving its major components and a greater semantic correspondence in the levels of abstraction emerging from the focal meanings.

INTERPRETIVE DIMENSION

The interpretive dimension is a process of crystallizing the meaning of the research findings. The researcher precisely illuminates the essential meaning of the findings through the articulation and discussion of the generated hypotheses. These hypotheses act as foci for the construction of theoretical and research structures and practice strategies. Andre's interpretation of the findings takes into consideration all of the phases of the research process through a logical progression. She relates the findings to the researcher's perspective, the method, and to nursing science. Andre links the four crucial elements of the general structural description for *reaching out* with Parse's principles. She contextualizes the phenomenon of *reaching out* as a pattern of interrelating in which one is unselfishly committed to another's welfare in a pushing-resisting process that requires energy and is ultimately transformed by an imaged or envisioned relationship which is confirming and subsequently revitalizing. Andre compares the theoretical conceptualizations set forth in the researcher's perspective with the findings of her study. This process may be viewed as an interpretive error, in that Spiegelberg's (1976) phenomenological research model proceeds from the lived experience of phenomena to abstract structures of meaning describing the experience. Rather than generate hypotheses that clearly emerge from the findings, Andre works to incorporate her findings into the theoretical conceptualizations described in the researcher's perspective. While it is appropriate to connect findings to the theoretical conceptualizations in the researcher's perspective, the findings in Andre's study do not clearly or consistently show the connections that she articulates. A purpose of nursing research is to enhance the developing body of nursing science by relating findings to theoretical perspectives and it is imperative that the researcher proceed strictly from the findings to congruent emergent theoretical structures that are subsequently related to extant nursing theory. For example, as Andre relates her findings to Parse's principles, she attempts to link the results to the concept of revealing-concealing appearing in the researcher's perspective; however, revealing-concealing does not clearly emerge from the findings. On the other hand, Andre's interpretation of the correspondence of the findings with the first principle of Man-Living-Health, although at times ambiguous, does represent an authentic relationship between findings and theory.

An alternate interpretation of the findings suggests the emergence of appropriate propositions. For example, the rhythm of pushing-resisting that occurs in *reaching out* places the subject in a highly vulnerable position in which the subject is faced with losing something in the relationship that is highly valued. The envisioned or imaged relationship guides the subject's growth toward interrelating in a particular way. This process required a determination on the part of each subject to stay with the envisioned relationship. Imaging the ultimate acceptance by the other in *reaching out* also appears to be essential to the transformation and energy mobilization that occurs.

An alternative theoretical proposition is: *reaching out* is a particular pattern of pushing-resisting in which one experiences a sense of vulnerability while pressing the other toward that which is not readily accepted by the other. This process is powered by imaging the ultimate acceptance by the other.

Andre's derivation of future research structures confirms this study's heuristic value. Andre suggests extending the scope of the study to include more subjects of different ages and genders. Two additional phenomenological studies related to the meaning of commitment were also discussed. The idea of commitment emerged in the general structural description of the phenomenon of *reaching out*, and is an appropriate focus for further research. Although Andre asked subjects to describe a situation of mutual *reaching out*, the focal meanings do not clearly reflect the subjects' descriptions of their experiences of another *reaching out* to them. By creating a phenomenological study focusing on the phenomenon of being reached out to, a separate and distinct perspective of the phenomenon of *reaching out* might be discovered. This would help to further explicate the mutual, simultaneous nature of Man–Man interrelationships. The case method might also be utilized to uncover the meaning of the experience of *reaching out*. For example, the researcher might develop categorical questions related to the findings of this study, such as, "When do you find yourself *reaching out* to another?" "What helps you continue to reach out to another?" "In what situations do you feel yourself *reaching out* to another?" This might further uncover the health experience as lived in the Man–Man interrelationship of *reaching out*.

In the interpretive dimension, the nurse researcher is responsible for specifying practice strategies suggested by the findings. Andre's recommendations for practice are rather nebulous, and do not offer distinct strategies for changing health patterns with families. Knowing that in the process of connecting with another in *reaching out* individuals will resist or push away from the other, the nurse illuminates the pattern, pushing-resisting, as generic to the powering process which exists in *reaching out*. The nurse helps the family members describe to each other what they want from each other. This is comparable to the "envisioned relationships" that emerged in Andre's findings. One way that the nurse synchronizes family energies is by reframing what might resemble a family battle in terms of an asynchronous rhythm of *reaching out*. The nurse may discuss with the family members the meaning of being engaged with each other in this way. Mobilization of energies is made possible through discovering the meaning of the relationships. Through illuminating patterns, synchronizing rhythms, and mobilizing energies, the nurse-family process propels the family toward revitalizing growth. Other practice strategies could be developed from the findings of this study.

As qualitative research continues to grow as a viable and necessary research approach for understanding health, it will be possible to relate a specific phenomenon, such as *reaching out*, to other empirically validated health phenomena. This study of the lived experience of *reaching out* is valuable for nursing science because it is a preliminary investigation of a specific phenomenon that occurs in patterns of interrelating that are dimensions of health.

APPENDIX A1
DESCRIPTIVE EXPRESSIONS

GROUP 1. ENERGY: INVIGORATING FORCE

Being at ease engaged in vigorous activity
Playing football
Eating good food and exercising
Feeling well
Ability to run and play free
Active and camping enjoying the sunshine and fresh air
Running, jumping, playing football
Feels good to run and jog
Participation in athletic events—running, jogging, tennis—
    especially outdoor activities
Feeling relaxed after a strenuous activity
Planning future goals for increasing activity
Running and playing
Feeling good after strenuous exercise
Eating good food
Exercising and lifting weights
Having fun in the playground
Playing basketball with my friends
Feeling happy and having fun in school
Eating and sleeping properly
Feeling that you can do anything
Feeling fit when training for a race
Running and sliding at basketball game
When first kissed my girlfriend
Feel I could do anything I wanted to
Playing football and jumping in the leaves
Running and playing football
Feeling optimistic
Training for track and field

Vitality; The most alive feeling I could imagine by getting fresh air
   and being able to go out and move around
Feeling good about yourself
Feeling good all the time
Feeling totally alive and full of energy while feeling great about
   everything and everybody
Enthusiastic
Positive outlook on all things
Feeling loose and active when doing exercises
Fun, nice, exciting
Feeling the fresh air while jogging and feeling really good
Feeling really good about the end of school and going to camp
Feeling good inside when riding a bike and playing
Establishing good health patterns
Feeling happy when jogging around the block
When I ride my bike, going up and down hills I feel glad
Trying out for cheerleading—warming up—made me feel good and
   alive
I feel good not having cookies and candy
Feeling really good having fun playing games (sports)
You can do more when you are feeling good
After jogging I feel so good. I could go on and on
Full of energy—ready for anything when I wash my hair—whole
   body feels bouncy
Being on vacation—running, jumping, flying, breathing fresh air
I feel I can do anything—even difficult tasks
Feeling physically fit is a good feeling
Feeling strong
Ability to be surprised with a gift
A good attitude about oneself
Feeling good all over about myself

GROUP 1. PLENTITUDE: CONSTRUCTING SUCCESSFULNESS

Having a well toned body
A job well done followed by easy relaxation
Feeling of satisfaction at accomplishing a goal
Having a sense of what the future holds
Improving one's technical skills; i.e., playing football better
Winning in competition with the best
Feeling of accomplishment
Winning a competitive meet

Good feelings associated with winning basketball games
Feel more creative and productive
Knowing that I am producing at my highest level
More capable at solving math problems
Accomplishing what I want
Leading the cheer leaders
I feel better about myself with a thinner and firmer body
While taking fitness test in gym.—I pushed myself beyond and felt
    good about myself
It felt great to know I completed the whole test.—top 40% of girls
    in U.S.A.
Finishing a race made me glad
Accomplishing something—like dancing which feels very good
Being able to do what I want to do with friends
Giving up something that is enjoyed for someone else and
    replacing personal benefits
Accomplishing a feat
Felt strong winning a race
A wholesome feeling about life which engenders confidence in
    one's ability to solve problems and cope with peer pressure
Increasing awareness of being able to risk so as to overcome the
    impossible
Ability to achieve the unexpected

GROUP 1. HARMONY: RESONATING CLARITY

Doing what one enjoys
When all is going well, life is lovely
Relief at hearing good news
Celebrating holidays with friends, family and good food
Doing what one wants to do
Going along as usual without thinking about how I feel
Sense of well-being
Camaraderie with others engaged in a similar activity
Assurance that one can walk and run after a crisis
Doing something you like to do; i.e., football
Receiving good reports
Vacationing with family
Being in control of your own life
Family getting along together
Doing well
Pleasure of being soaking wet and then getting dry

Clear fresh sunny spring morning
Feeling nervous then anxious then comfortable when debating
Enjoying debating with others
Enjoyable feeling of inspiration
Free state of being
Health is taking care of yourself with care
Getting presents on your birthday; being with family
Happy and pain free
Being with my family shopping and picking out neat outfits
Being with others
Happy, relaxed, relieved
Freedom and independence; well-being with happiness
Having someone there when you hurt
Feeling happy
Having fun with friends, getting tired and going home
Feel in control and strong
Feeling together—after I swim—with sunshine on my face
Relief at hearing good news
Feeling of health is like a spring morning—cool, breezy and sunny
Having freedom and enjoying the things I like to do
Traveling with friends
Feeling of (relief) happy
Feeling of health is being relaxed, having self confidence I can
    accomplish more
Being with others for a celebration
Happy running along with my Mom
Health is when I'm peaceful and happy in a warm caring
    atmosphere
Mentally sharp, physically calm with self and others
Being with friends who value what you say
Unforgettable feeling of relief after pain subsides
Being free from worry and disease
Walking and riding a bike; listening to music, dancing, playing
    violin
Meeting new friends and playing football with them

APPENDIX A2
DESCRIPTIVE EXPRESSIONS

GROUP 2. ENERGY: SPIRITED INTENSITY

Energetic
Enthusiastic
Desire to eat more nourishing food improved appearance
Felt very energetic and exuberant while walking
Feel healthy physically, mentally, emotionally
Excited about feeling good and looking good
Perceive things in a positive manner
Able to sustain pain and fatigue
At least 6 hours of sleep
Eating well balanced meals
Participating vigorously in physical exercise
Catching a second wind
Waking up good and refreshed
Regular diet and exercise
Good nights sleep
Anticipated the day
Energy level high
General sense of well-being—feeling energetic
Positive outlook on life
Feel happy and strong like I could do anything I wanted to
Jogging regularly
Feeling good about self
Being full of energy and not tired
Feeling skinny and good about myself
Great feeling of diving into a swimming pool
Feeling good and happy
Exercising and walking
Feeling good each morning
Dieting and jogging every day
Excitement, anticipation and good will

Riding against the wind, tingly, awake, and ready for the day
Feeling full of energy
Looking forward
Energy to move, think and feel better
Feeling good all over
Participating in sports
Aware of how well I felt
Thinking how great to be alive happy and loved
Feeling like I'm king of the world and nothing can bother me
Being in on exercise program
Energetic
Feel in peak condition
Good all around attitude
Positive attitude about self
Playing basketball
Stretching and running
Feeling good
Biking in a state park
Feeling good about self
Feeling of refreshment
Feeling good about the world
Strong and anxious to go on living
Looking forward with hope to a fulfilling future
A glowing light of energy burning brightly in my eyes
Experiencing life to the fullest
Hypnotic relaxed feeling while running
Strong and healthy
Hiking trip to Smoky Mountains
Tired but exhilarated
Feel alert and refreshed
Overall satisfied healthy feeling
A whip the world feeling
Using muscle and brains for a full days work
Strenuous physical work
After running and stretching—state of euphoria and well-being
While running had more strength
Feeling good
Feeling control over body while jogging
Surge of energy
Overall feeling of well-being
More energy to take on tasks
Functioning completely
Feeling fit while engaged in dancing program

Feeling positive about looks
Feeling glowing and most independent
Feeling strength and exhilaration
A sense of renewal after running
Reflection on how good it is to be alive
A new feeling of being good all over
Feel energetic
Think clearly
A positive mental attitude about body
Belief that I could do or be anything I wanted
Increased strength
Feeling really good
A beautiful feeling
Feeling renewed and strong
Thoughts of longer life while exercising
Feeling of strength and versatility
Exercising
Feeling of exhilaration
Feeling proud of myself while exercising
Feeling of alertness and purpose—looking forward to the day
Feeling both exhausted and exhilarated when running
Waking up fresh, awake and alive
Exhilaration and personally challenging while skiing and back
     packing
Pushing a little extra and being enthusiastic
After physical exercise or walk on beach
Walking every day
Feeling good about self
While running through woods body awakens and awareness
     blooms to a euphoric plateau.
After jogging feel loose and a desire for work
Participating in school activities
Feeling great

GROUP 2. PLENTITUDE: FULFILLING INVENTIVENESS

Tolerate stress
Finishing a project that takes up time—feeling accomplished
Motivated to keep going on
Accomplishing physical tasks
Feeling reassured of capabilities
Trying some new endeavor

Focus on things other than constant stress
Personal achievement and sense of accomplishment
Feeling good about losing weight
Feeling there was more of life that could be enjoyed
Feeling good because of dieting and losing weight
Feeling like a new person when losing weight
Dieting and knowing I am losing weight
Lucky that I was healthy enough to participate in physical
    education course
A slim body
Sweating and pushing body
Attain goals that I set for self
Accomplishing something
Body performing perfectly
Accomplishing going beyond the barrier of starting and continuing
    the run
Doing a good job and feeling good about self
Accomplishment
Exceed over stress
Vigorous training to put me in the best shape of my life
Accomplishing as much as I can
Feeling satisfied that my job was completed well
Good feeling and accomplishment to take care of self
Feeling and accomplishing something positive in enriching my life
Able to overcome a problem
Completing an exercise program
Ability to extend the limits of endurance
Continuing on a regular schedule
Could play racket ball for an hour and not be exhausted
Satisfying feeling of accomplishment after a strenuous task
Feeling of being reborn and given another chance
A growing confidence in physical abilities on long bicycle trip
Feeling of accomplishment while running
A sense of achievement
Feel successful as a person
Awareness of activity level associated with completing a difficult
    task
Able to care for self
A challenge
Staying in shape
Winning the game of life
Resumption of routine activities
A feeling of freedom and self fulfillment on developing own
    corporation

Teaching—doing what I struggled for
Knowing that I am doing something great for the body
Noticing ease of bending, flexing and jumping because of exercise
    program
Feeling of accomplishment
Accomplishing things quickly and satisfactorily
Accomplishing a challenging hike
Still able to keep up in comparison with others
Conflict about commitment while moving
Knowing that body shape is getting better

GROUP 2. HARMONY: SYMPHONIC INTEGRITY

Entire person spiritual, physical & mental
Balance of parts
Health impacts life, family and environment
A state of healthiness vs unhealthiness
Require less rest
Rested and at ease
Balanced academic and social life
Feel tired but aware that muscles are in good shape
No aches or pains
Happy and confident about how day would go
Felt relaxed and clean physically and emotionally
Fun and time shared with healthy people
Peaceful attitude
Enjoying self
Overall well-being
Crisp clean air
Relaxed
Nothing hurts
Feeling of a good self image and that the others loved me—feeling
    of worth
Sorting through daily activities
Confident in self, happy and cheerful
Feeling a glow around my world, a sound view
Free of self conscious thoughts—being myself
Not judging others or being judged by others
Feeling sad and depressed at the death of a loved one yet thankful
    at being healthy and alive
Feelings of loneliness and depression would be lessened in the
    presence of others
Doing something positive for self

Like ice cream—nice and cool
A peaceful feeling inside when bicycling
Enjoying own space at that moment
Getting wrapped up in my world
Thoughts going off into peaceful and alone feelings
Noticing the world around me
Mind becomes tranquil
Take off leaving all worries and strains of life behind
Happiness associated with the return of a loved one
Perceiving world as a neat place
More comfortable and secure
Keenly aware of Spring
Pleasant warm breeze
Drinking in the beauty of the day
Just right feeling about everything
Breathing fresh air
Not feeling tired, lazy or sick
Being in the ocean breeze with sun rays beating down
Nowhere to be or nothing to do
No worries or work to do
Relaxed
Mind at ease and clear
Peace of mind
Feeling of well-being
Rhythmical, easy and warm
Like a fine piece of machinery—clear head and could think
Feeling of being in control
When pregnant
Glowing and good inside
Privileged, happy and special
Feeling the baby kick
Not having to go to work or school
Shining sun
Questioning about meaning of work and anxiety
Well being and comfortableness of knowing self
Breathing fresh air and using muscles
Happy, warm and relaxed
Peaceful
Good tired feeling
Physical and mental well-being
At peace with those I care about and myself
Mind being free and clear of all activities while looking at fire
Body functioning at slowest pace

Every part of body totally relaxed
Nothing hurts
Beautiful sunny day
Contented; a feeling of well-being
Sleep a little later and go for a walk
Breathe quite deeply
Muscles feel loose and used
Mental and physical well-being
Assuming responsibility for self
Felt more at ease
Balance and integration of self as whole
Less subject to frustration
Breathed better
A heightening of ego
Taking responsibility for own health
Enjoying children as they laugh, jump, play
Giving, taking, caring, and struggle of life
Being together with family and feeling strong
Confident and self assured
Less anxious
Feeling of control of health and source of comfort and
      contentment
Appreciating God
Questioning bodily feelings after strenuous exercise
A calm seemed to pervade my being after stopping smoking and
      taking up racquet ball
More comfortable with self at work and in social situations
Clear mind
Fresh smelling air
Good happy thoughts
Being cared for
Contentment
Happiness
Feeling loved
Peace of mind
Feel one with body
Being thankful for good health when watching handicapped people
Freedom of mind and body while engaged in sports
A focus on a particular moment
Feeling ebb and flow with the goal
Feeling at ease after completing Fall semester
Kind to everyone
Relief

Improved confidence
Relief, mind at ease
Feeling of freedom
Playing with son
Inner sense of tranquility and harmony associated with excess
    physical activity
Awe struck and at peace with my existence
Pleasantly exhausted
More aware of body
A sense of everything working well
Pressures and concerns of previous days seemed much less
World and cares seem far away
Feeling of contentment, love and happiness after moving into
    fiancee's apartment
Happier with self and world
More aware of surroundings
Increased self esteem
Awareness of bodily change
No demands or obstacles

GROUP 3. ENERGY: EXHILARATED POTENCY

I had a clear headed, clear mind and energy restored
Felt I could lick the world
I had a lot of energy
I felt good all over, lots of happy thoughts
I felt extra good and alert after a good nights sleep
Laughing, singing and enjoying exercises to music
Energy surging through my body.
Wonderful feeling of being alive. I'm glad I am Me.
Feeling good about self, what and who one is
Keeping active and interested
Feeling of strength
Great feeling on hearing good news
Active engagement in daily activity
I feel alert with all my sensory perceptions functioning at high
    gear.
Having the energy to do the activities you want to do
Keeping busy with housework and hobbies; i.e., reading and crafts
Being eager to face life
Felt fresh, well-rested and glad to be alive
I feel really good involved in active, strenuous exercise
Active participation in keeping fit
Vitality and energy of a physical endeavor
Desire to take better care of self
Having strength to work all day without pain
A sense of energy
Eager upon arising
Energetic most of the day
My mood was usually cheerful, enthusiastic; observed objectively
    by friends, relatives as looking so well
Feeling good about not having problems that can't be handled

Awareness of active participation in remaining healthy
Heightened awareness of sense perception—glad to be alive—
    thinking, moving, experiencing
Active participation in keeping well through exercise
Keeping active and being involved with people each day.
Engaging in sports and enjoying higher levels of energy
Ability to go anywhere and do anything I wanted to do
A feeling of total well-being
Overall feeling of well-being from engaging in vigorous physical
    activity and proper rest
A good feeling all over on engaging in vigorous activity
A positive outlook toward life and day to day living
Ability to work and perform all other activities
I experience health when engaged in physical exercise such as
    walking or cutting wood
Feeling great from involvement in vigorous activity
Feeling good everyday is a feeling of health
Feeling positive about life
Feeling of self-renewal
Engaged in yard work
Feels good just to be alive
Getting up each morning and functioning throughout the day
Feeling that I can handle anything that comes along
Health is a positive feeling of all-around well-being
Walking fast
Distinct feeling of increased alertness
Shocking awareness of one's mortality
I was strong, having mastered the wind and storm and met life
    head on—I had never felt so well.
A sense of being glad to be alive and pain-free
Health is in feeling there aren't enough hours in the day to work—
    having barrels of energy fighting to get out
A good feeling about feeling good.

GROUP 3. PLENTITUDE: CREATING TRIUMPHS

Ability to meet criticism and adverse circumstances
Ability to cope with any problems
Satisfaction of a goal accomplished and its special memories
Achievement of many life goals
Having a good marriage and watching children grow up
Ability to do a job

Sense of well-being in having accomplished something
Having goals, good attitudes of accomplishments
Feeling of having accomplished the daily work load
Doing for self and others
Sense of accomplishment at moving through a daily routine
    smoothly
Ability to take care of home and also work
Ability to do what I'd planned
Felt good at completion of a task
Accomplishment felt in a thing well done in an easy, unhurried
    outing with a friend
Successful conclusion of a stressful situation
Capable of accomplishing anything I wanted to do
Pride and joy in accomplishing what I want to do
Ability to achieve a goal
Ability to be productive
A day with things to do and plans to be made
Having a plan for the future but living one day at a time to its
    fullest
Feeling of accomplishment
Overcoming adversity
Feeling of well-being in overcoming crises
Pride in accomplishing planned activities and work
Feeling relief and pride at having risked and succeeded.
Feeling that there is no challenge one cannot meet
Being involved with less fortunate others. Making life progressive
    and useful by having projects to complete
Being able to do and enjoy the activities of the day is a feeling of
    health
Being able to do things I like to do to help others and keep up with
    responsibility
Feeling of self-satisfaction and fulfillment

GROUP 3. HARMONY: SERENE UNITY

Feeling of physical and mental well-being
Knowledge of what is to happen
General sense of everything's right
No ache—pain—no nausea—no tension; frees you to think about
    other things
General sense of everything's right
Physical, mental, and social well-being

Completely at peace with myself, family and environment
Feel free of pain, depression or aches
I have peace of mind
I'm free to do as I like
Enjoying retirement and the presence of children, grandchildren
    and friends
Internal "glow" shown in lovely lustrous hair
Thinking good thoughts and put your trust in the Lord
Opportunity to be free, open and expressive with friends
Creation of the spirit of peace, calm and belonging
Sense of getting in touch with my deepest central self—enjoyed
    the sunsets and sunrise
Opportunity for quiet time with the Lord
Uncluttered mind, clear focus, love and acceptance
Feeling of wholeness and complete
Times of sharing with husband, children and friends
Feeling of one with the environment
Thinking happy thoughts
Feeling of peace with life and surroundings
Sense of relationship with environment
Thinking happy thoughts
Feeling of peace with life and surroundings
Sense of relationship with environment
Health means happiness
Feeling of relief on hearing good news
Rested feeling that promotes daily activities
Self-confidence
Feeling of peace with the environment
A pleasant afternoon with family
Health means to me—keeping active and being happy, physically
    and mentally
Joy at seeing husband feeling better following an illness
Discomfort in the plight of another and grateful for own good
    health
Feeling of well-being; i.e., work long hours in the yard, take long
    walks
Walking on the beach—a feeling of unhurried freedom, no
    pressures
Being one with the world of nature—a part of the universe
Feeling light inside, relaxed in mind and body, joyous
To be able to walk, see the world around us touch our loved ones,
    smell the roses, etc.
Successful relationships

Enjoyment of every day as a wonderful, beautiful experience

Satisfying interpersonal relationships with co-workers, family and
friends

Feeling of well-being even in situations with large possibilities

Restful sleep

A clean environment in which to awaken each morning

An uncluttered day

Health is each person's responsibility for his own well-being

Growing awareness of own responsibility in health practice

Freedom from pressures and overbearing demands

Continuing feeling of well-being over time

Commitment to practice better health activities

Growing awareness of own participation in feeling good

Complete state of being in which one achieves physical-mental
and social equilibrium

Interaction with others in social intercourse

Ability to be one with the world

Feelings of freedom from pain and unhappiness

Increasing awareness of own responsibility and accountability for
health practices

Contradictory feelings of pride, gratitude, yet nagging fear of what
the future holds

A clear mind, a joyful heart and a body devoid of upset and hurt is
my experience of health

Confidence in knowing that there is life beyond the grave

Opportunity to explore different perspectives of life

The opportunity to live each day is an experience of health

Appreciation of own health in confronting others' serious
problems.

Health is seizing the opportunities that life extends; i.e.,
happiness and the privilege of education

Having and enjoying pleasant company; i.e., wife, children and
parents

Sensation of increased relaxation and comfort on daily run

Increasing awareness of one's own power

Realization that feelings of loneliness are conquered within oneself
and not from outside

Growing awareness of need to assume responsibility for health
practices.

A feeling of sharpened sensitivity in all senses and a more
insightful perspective

Feeling one with the environment; i.e., the smell of the woods,
the crunching of leaves underfoot crowds out the tensions of
the day

A sense of relaxation in the experience of a change in day to day
   routines
Health is being happy
Health is an expression of love to family and other loved ones
Health is like floating on air
Ability to feel in control of one's life
Opportunity to be independent and active
A certain serenity
A sense of being in control
Harmonious relationship with others
Observed objectively by friends, relatives as looking well
A sense of closeness to God.

APPENDIX A4
DESCRIPTIVE EXPRESSIONS

GROUP 4. ENERGY: TRANSCENDENT VITALITY

You feel so good when you're healthy
You feel like getting out and jumping around
Positive outlook important
I exercise a lot—am in good health
Being healthy is being able to do anything you want to do
Back to H.S. after retirement, recalling wonderful things, I became
   renewed in body and mind—I wanted to see and remember
   everything
Renewal, alive-well—joy within me and a more positive view of
   life.
I feel as I did 30 years ago—go shopping, play bridge, go to lunch
   with friends
Most health after daily exercise and meditation; I get a new
   outlook on life and new energy for my activities
Grateful for vitality to continue doing things taken for granted in
   youth
Walk with zest admiring surroundings we took for granted.
Fun to walk through mall just to look instead of dashing to select
   an article
Realizing that others can't get around as you do you say "I feel
   great"!
Long distance bike ride—good feeling of health
Do many physical activities such as biking, hiking, dancing with
   no ill effects
I hope to continue this way
Good outlook on life
Steps were light, I felt tall, far above my troubles. (When I feel
   well those are my tall days)
Feeling good and so happy to be normal and alive like I was
Others so kind I feel I can get up and go again

Feeling good is feeling healthy

I felt refreshed and good in care of others

Feeling of physical emotional and mental well-being that enables me to go about daily routine with enthusiasm

When I wake up in the morning rested and think of what a beautiful morning—then get up and attack whatever needs to be done with gusto

Great wonderful feeling—health

On lovely day I experience feeling of euphoria and am thankful for health

To feel good enough to do what's necessary, gardening—turns me on

I played, all kinds of athletics, active outdoors

I have the heart and lungs of a 50-year-old person—I go to health spa to exercise and whirlpool 3 times a week

Golfing, swimming, gardening give me a feeling of exhilaration and at the same time tranquility

Went to work after surgery

I joined a square dance club for seniors and that really is an experience of health as I feel young and it's really exercising

Being able to sleep and wake up refreshed

Meeting with family for happy music—I danced and acted silly—like my old self

Persistent good feeling

Feeling good reminds me of childhood, a surge of energy, work and relaxation

40 years of good health, could do anything—whatever was needed could do

Feel good

Exercise everyday

Positive thinking

Positive attitude necessary

Feel fine zest for life, feel same as when I was 30—physically and mentally

Feel good all over—you don't know what tired is—go-go-go

Feel vibrant and full of zip—you're healthy

When I get up in morning and feel good enough to do my normal duties of the day—all of my own maintenance and then go out dancing

To be able to eat well—bowl—drive, think young

Kids on picnic keep me young—seeing others, vibrant and enthusiastic about life is catching, makes me feel so healthy and alive, good times

Feeling fit, unusually energetic as though I could accomplish
  anything I tried to do
Enjoy life when able to garden, and maintain house; hope to
  continue to do so
When able to feed cattle, do chores and raise garden
Keeping active and enjoying hobbies
I feel best when doing something physical like walking briskly,
  bicycling or working in yard; aches and pains go and head is
  clear
Would like to go on living for a long time
Attending health spa often
Feeling fine
Feeling pretty good—hoping to stay that way in the future
Being able to carry on work as a farmer
Feeling good without problems
Enjoyed excellent feeling
Elated with ability to maneuver about the mountains
Physically tired—I felt very good and exhilarated
Feeling strong, exercising
Able to do physical labor
Feeling of aliveness
Stronger and fit for battle of life after minor setback
Feeling great and enjoying life to its fullest
Encountering others strongly giving fellow man a hard time as
  long as I can
I look forward to future—not back
Positive attitude
Wonderful feeling of well-being
Having a vast supply of energy
Feeling euphoric on brighter clear crisp day, think cheery, tolerant
  and make decisions
Good mental outlook
No task seemed too difficult
Square dancing, I love life
I feel good

GROUP 4. PLENTITUDE: GENERATING COMPLETENESS

Drive by myself—out west
Now for my grandson I do housework, laundry, prepare meals.
When able to function independently I can care for personal
  happiness, physical care and keep yards in order, shop, visit
  friends

Working—health when I was younger taking care of family, feeling
rested and feeling good about completing my work

Live every day to fullest not thinking of future

I feel health now after open heart surgery; I never smoked and
don't drink beer.

Able to accomplish extensive household tasks in one day

Capable of functioning with most of today's perplexing problems
and know when to hang on and when to let go

The joy and appreciation of being able to read and drive make life
worth living

When I was able to work all day, care for children, dig in garden

Being able to perform my duties

Not tired and the ability to do little jobs or tasks

I experience good health and happiness after painting a picture; a
combination of physical and mental energy and creative
activity

A feeling of good health comes to me when I look at a pile of
firewood—the results of my labor from felling the tree to the
finished product.

Can do regular work

Immense satisfaction in working with people who need assistance

Healthy attitude for work—appreciate physical, mental abilities
required to study long hrs. to comprehend laws to help clients

Looking from golf course over Pacific Ocean with an 85 for 18—
feel really good

Doing something that requires physical and mental activity and
gives a feeling of accomplishment

Participation in productive activities

Brightness of day shone in completion of studies

New me felt I could complete all plans on time

Being able to participate and achieve my goals

Feel relaxed knowing I tried to help others enjoy life by being a
good example to youngsters

Full day's work, no disabilities

Being able to travel

GROUP 4. HARMONY: SYNCHRONOUS CONTEMPLATION

Health is well-being

You don't have different aches and pains

Just living where the air is fresh and clear, good water, lots of
space for a garden is enough to create in one a sense of good
health

Good neighbors, churches and schools contribute to good state of
  mental health
Healthy when someone talks to me
Enjoying good health is most important next to God
Health problems are taken care of by God, doctors and love of
  husband and family
Feeling of health comes from real peace of mind brought about
  only by making decisions and sticking to them
I visited the violet patch where wild flowers grew—stopped at the
  stables where cows and horses were kept, visited chapel
When I go to see my son and granddaughter
Feeling of good health most important to enjoyment
Relief and joy felt after being told good news
Blest with good health
Having faith in God and complete trust in doctors takes away
  anxious feelings
To be free of anything which would alter my optimum
  functioning, my well-being or progress
I feel happy, peace of mind, comfort, joy when free from worry of
  not being independent and able to make own decision
Youth takes health for granted
Health is riches, proper diet, exercise, everything in moderation
You can't buy health—hold on to it, appreciate it
Travel extensively seeing new places—revisiting old places
Remain active in moderate social life with husband
Knowledge and information about health practices
Absence of pain after gall bladder removal
Felt like a new person after control of health problems
Awareness of passage of time fades away, relaxed, free of anxiety,
  experiencing pleasurable almost mystical activation of mind
Drawing and painting seem to bring the physical, mental and
  emotional together in a relaxed, pleasurable, unsurpassed state
  of well-being
Health is God given
I enjoyed my family; they are loving children
Generalized, sense of feeling the best over time—now slowing
  down
Like a bright sunny day in May when all is right with God and my
  fellow men
Not feeling helpless
I enjoy being with people
Feeling of thankfulness to God—appreciation that I live in modern
  times with health technologies
Being able to breath easily

Free from aches and pain
Wondering how various situations would affect well-being
Family glad to see me—I was feeling pretty good
Having people loving me and caring for me
Getting rest—being free of exhaustion and insecurity
Taking interest in care of the house—more relaxed
Enjoy dogs, keeping busy
Free of aches or pain to do what I want to do—go anywhere—a
    dance—and play cards
When outside—as a kid I'll run through woods, run a wheel on the
    road or wrestle with a friend
Warm outside—sun made me feel warm all over
I was walking around my house smelling good air, I felt good
After retirement I felt health—free to go my own way—no bills—I
    built my own house free and clear of debt.
Thank God for strength and ability to enjoy working and living an
    active life
When I have little pain and financial and other problems
No aches and pain, feel good
I don't want others to take care of you. I like to be around people
    to talk and help others
To arise to morning feeling fully rested and no pains and aches
I don't worry about tomorrow, just live for today
Sense of well-being
I feel well as my friends say I look
Living without focusing on health as a consideration
Freedom from worry
Secure feeling—feeling of being well and cared for—with access to
    help from professionals
Being free of apprehension
Walking, looking, listening to the woods sounds that reminded me
    of another life time
Thankful for care
Not being depressed
A feeling of well-being knowing that He was with me
Being all right
Thank God for good feeling
Not having exhausted feeling or being dependent on others
Making the best of what is
Enjoy many activities in retirement within limitations
Able to have enjoyable intimate relationship with wife
Freedom from encumbrance
Optimum feeling of health occurs while I'm painting or drawing

Appendix B1

First Level Analysis: 18 Domains; Representing 7 Different Universal
Semantic Relationships

DOMAINS	UNIVERSAL SEMANTIC RELATIONSHIPS
1. Ways to get through the day	X is a way to do Y (means-end)
2. Kinds of problems	X is a kind of Y (strict inclusion)
3. Kinds of relationships	X is a kind of Y (strict inclusion)
4. Ways to create privacy	X is a way to do Y (means-end)
5. Ways to avoid getting lost	X is a way to do Y (means-end)
6. Kinds of persons	X is a kind of Y (strict inclusion)
7. Reasons for going along	X is a reason for Y (rationale)
8. Places for recreation	X is a place for Y (location for action)
9. Steps to getting adjusted	X is a step (stage) in Y (sequence)
10. Places to get bathed	X is a place for Y (location for action)
11. Characteristics of nurses	X is a characteristic of Y (attribution)
12. Characteristics of the home	X is a characteristic of Y (attribution)
13. Kinds of meals	X is a kind of Y (strict inclusion)
14. Ways to get family to visit	X is a way to Y (means-end)
15. Reasons for getting hair done	X is a reason for Y (rationale)
16. Kinds of fears	X is a kind of Y (strict inclusion)
17. Places in the home	X is a part of Y (spatial)
18. Parts of the room	X is a part of Y (spatial)

DOMAINS SELECTED FOR IN-DEPTH ANALYSIS WITH INCLUDED TERMS

Domain: *Ways to get through the day*
Included Terms: doing activities
                       looking at T.V.
                       eating
                       napping
                       casual talking
                       remembering better times
                       pretending you're at home
                       waiting for visitors
                       waiting for medicine
                       waiting to die
                       trying to keep busy

Domain: *Kinds of Problems*
Included Terms: falling asleep
                       dying alone-not being found
                       limited personal space
                       friends all gone
                       being lonely
                       all dressed up and no place to go
                       becoming a burden
                       put "away" from center of things
                       no good for anything
                       people (nurses) lie to you
                       whole way of life changes
                       can't walk or see or even eat anymore

Domain: *Kinds of Relationships*
Included Terms: best foot forward
                       waiting (for nothing)
                       being a "pet"
                       "polite talking"
                       nothing to say
                       learning to be alone
                       keeping other residents distant so you don't lose
                           again
                       being close but not too close

Domain: *Ways to create privacy*
Included Terms: draw curtain
                       turn chair away
                       go to lounge
                       try to have lunch
                       pretend to nap
                       pretend to look at T.V.
                       read
                       take a walk

Domain: *Kinds of fear*
Included Terms: being helpless
                       winding up like them (those in skilled care
                           nursing home)
                       falling
                       breaking bones
                       having a stroke
                       having to be force fed
                       going blind
                       being deaf
                       not being able to care for self
                       having to depend on others

Appendix B3

Taxonomy for the Domain: Ways to Get Through the Day

Doing activities	Routine	Current Events Bingo Horseshoes
	Special	Holiday Parties Sing-a-long Birthday parties Pet Day (dogs & cats)
Looking at TV		
Eating	Meals	Breakfast Dinner Supper
	Snacks	Evening before bed
	Treats	Parties
		Special Visiting groups Holidays
Napping		
Casual Talking	Roommate	Roommate's family Roommate's visitors
	Staff Workers	Nurses Secretaries Nurses' aides Beautician
	Other people	Laundry Kitchen Office Janitor
Remembering Better Times	School days	High school beaus College chums Nice teachers
	Work Being a bride Having children Spouse living Vacations with family	
	Feeling better	Could see Could hear Go anywhere Do anything
	Cooking	
	Happy times	Spouse alive Caring for children Birth of grandchildren Visiting family & friends
	Sad times	Parents' death Husband's death Money problems Illnesses Out of work

TAXONOMY FOR THE DOMAIN: WAYS TO GET THROUGH THE DAY—*Continued*

Pretending you're still in your own home

Waiting for Visitors	Family	
	Friends	
	People from church	
	School children	
	Pet society with animals	
Waiting for medicine	Everyday ones	
	Special ones for pain	
Waiting to die	Nothing to do anymore	
	Lived too long	
	Sick and helpless	
	Alone	
	Burden to everyone	
Trying to keep busy	Fill the day	Reading
		Doing crafts
	Trying to feel useful	Help nurses fill pitchers
		Reading to residents who can't
		Help nurses fold linen

Appendix B4

Taxonomy for Domain: Ways to Get Through the Day
Componential Analysis

	DIMENSIONS OF CONTRAST			
CONTRAST SET	THINGS YOU CAN CONTROL	THINGS YOU HAVE TO BE CAREFUL ABOUT	HOLDS SOME DEGREE OF INTEREST	MAKES YOU FEEL CARED ABOUT
Looking at TV	Yes	No	Yes	Not really
Casual talking with nurse	No	Yes	No	No
Doing special activities	Yes	No	Yes	Yes
Daytime napping	Yes	No	—	—
Going to bed	No	—	—	—
Waiting to die	—	—	Nothing to do	—

HYPOTHETICAL PROPOSITIONS WITH SUPPORTING FIELD NOTES

Hypothetical Proposition 1

RARE MOMENTS OF REBELLIOUSNESS BEAR WITNESS TO THE QUIESCENT RAGE OF THE OLD.

Mrs. A

Mrs. A is a 78-year-old widow who is now residing in Nursing Home B. She has no children and her family and most of her friends are "gone." She describes herself as a nonconformist who would rather be "anywhere but here." She walks with the aid of a walker and although she is able to care for herself, she cannot manage to live alone. She presently occupies a private room but still experiences the situation as a surrender of her privacy. Even when she retreats to her room, staff and other residents generally walk in without knocking regardless of whether the door is open or closed. She has repeatedly asked "everyone" to please knock and for a few days, they do—but soon, they're back to just walking in. One morning I went in to find Mrs. A sitting in the hall outside the dining room on the first floor. She informed me that we would have to talk here rather than go upstairs to her room because she was being "punished." She said she did not know why she was being punished nor how long she would have to sit in the hall, but she would not "give them the satisfaction of asking." Throughout this exchange with me, Mrs. A chose her words very carefully and lowered her tone or stopped talking entirely when a staff person walked by. She glanced from side to side, her words coming in a sharp, clipped vibrato that could have been anger or the attempt to hold back tears—or both. I asked her how this made her feel and she responded in a voice very close to tears—"like a little child—I'm 78 years old and I'm trembling like a child—well, if they treat me like a child, I'll just act like one." Her way of being in this infantalizing situation was to refuse to eat or bathe and yet, she sat obediently in the assigned chair.

Mr. B

Mr. B comes to the elder center three to four times a week "to have lunch—play a little cards—talk—what else can an old man do?" He laughs when he says that "nobody wants you when you're old," he becomes very serious when he says he comes to the center "to get out of their [family] way." With a twinkle in his eye, he said that sometimes he leaves home and doesn't even tell his family he's leaving: After all, he's "not a baby." He says "That shakes them up a little," but he doesn't do it too often because he doesn't want them to put him "in a home."

Mr. & Mrs. C

Mr. and Mrs. C live in the home where they reared their five children. All children now live independently from the parental home. Two of the daughters live close by and the others live within 100–300 miles. The two daughters have become increasingly concerned that "The house is too much for Ma." They have begun to visit or call quite frequently. Much love and mutual concern is apparent . . . Mr. C told me he wished that the girls would not be such "clucking hens." Mrs. C joined in and laughingly agreed that she would "just like to lock the door on them." When I asked what this (locking the door) would represent, Mrs. C said that it made her "mad to be checked on like a kid."

Hypothetical Proposition II

PATTERNS OF INTERRELATING MAKE MANIFEST THE AUTOMATIC SURREALISM OF THE MEANINGLESS WORLDS OF THE OLD.

Mrs. D

Staff persons in the nursing homes create an illusion of cure which distances the residents and affirms the surrealistic ambience of the setting. Mrs. D is 80 years old and has "terminal cancer." She is described by the staff as "depressed because she is not getting better as fast as she should do so she can go home." When I asked Nurse O if Mrs. D would indeed get better and go home, she replied: "Oh, no, her prognosis is just weeks, but we can't let her think that—it would take away all her hope." In conversation with Mrs. D, she indicated that she knows she will never get better and go home. She knows she is, in fact, dying and perhaps this is best for she will no longer be a burden to anyone. Her "depression" seemed to be related more to the unreal atmosphere engendered in the illusion of cure.

Mrs. E

Mrs. E attends the elder center one to two times a week. She says her life has changed since she "can't get around as good" anymore. She misses her busy life but "you're better off with those your own age— young people—they don't want old fogies around." At the center, she works with ceramic crafts and says she "makes gifts for my friends that they probably put in the attic"—but—well, it "passes the day . . . and I meet nice people."

Mrs. F

Mrs. F lives with her granddaughter and husband and their children. The great grandchildren show much love for their great grandmother and have, in fact, become "protective" of her since "her mind began to slip." When the great grandchildren were small, Grandmother took care of them since both parents work outside the home. Mrs. F says she is now the one who needs a "babysitter" and she wonders out loud that "if another baby came," she could again "do something useful." She says she doesn't like T.V., so does a lot of "just sitting around."

Hypothetical Proposition III

THE THOUGHT OF PERSONAL DEATH LIES ALWAYS JUST AT THE SURFACE OF THE EXPLICIT.

Mrs. G

Mrs. G sleeps on a couch in the entry lounge of the nursing home. The nurse said that it's because her roommate is too noisy. Mrs. G told me she sleeps in the lounge because "they never come to your room at night unless you call them—what if something happened—they wouldn't even know it 'til morning."

Mrs. H

Mrs. H's daughter brings her to day care each day on her way to work. Although Mrs. H has some difficulty getting around, she really could stay home alone. In discussing this with Mrs. H, she said that she would rather stay at home but she comes to day care because "if anything happened," she wouldn't be found until her daughter came home in the evening.

Mr. I

Mr. I in describing Thanksgiving dinner says in a rather sober, pensive tone, "I've been cooking the holiday dinner for—I don't know how many years—and this was the first year I had to call for help to lift the bird out of the oven—I suppose that's what happens when you get old—I'll be 90 soon, you hear—maybe—next year—I won't have to lift it at all."

APPENDIX C

CASE STUDY INTERVIEW DATA

Interviewer What did you think of retirement before you retired. How did you think it would be?

Mr. E. Well, what I heard a lot of people say if you don't have any hobbies, don't retire. But people seem to retire as soon as they can. It's nothing but a rat race. But myself, as far as what I thought, I would have stayed longer, I could have stayed longer, but my leg and hip was giving me so much trouble I could not stand anymore. I decided I was 65 1/2 and took my retirement and have really enjoyed it so far.

Interviewer So then you decided to retire.

Mr. E. Yes, a year before I decided to retire my leg started hurting real bad and I went for X-rays, the doctor said my hip looked terrible from the time before.

Interviewer How about you, Mrs. E., what did you think about before you retired?

Mrs. E. Well, I really was not of age to retire. I was 59 when I quit work. I was working in a department store and the boss's wife she started giving everybody a hard time and I thought I would quit and I really looked forward to retiring. I've worked since I was in high school at different jobs and really never kept a permanent job. Then I kept this job for 12 years. The driving was getting monotonous. Twenty miles down and twenty miles back. I could have seen about another job, but when you have to travel to work when you are older you just, I don't know, toward the last I got so bored traveling back and forth. Then you were on your feet all day and stood all the time. It was getting tiresome.

Interviewer As you look back on your choice what stands out as being most important to you?

Mr. E. Well, that I would not have any more hassle. As far as the work, I liked it. I like being around people. It was too hard for me to stand and work, it would not have benefited me. I do miss the people.

Mrs. E. I think it was the thing I wanted to do and couldn't do before. I was on a time schedule. Get up at a certain time, come home at a certain time. I had meals to get. In the eve-

	ning I was doing the dishes at 7 o'clock and the evening was gone. I did not have any enjoyment. Now we are together more and you can go places and do things. If you want to go on trips, you just have more time and no limits.
Mr. E.	We get to go together a good bit and we could not do that before.
Mrs. E.	It wasn't that I had so much to do with a new home, there is not that much to do. But you are tired when you get home after working 8 hours and being on your feet and legs. I looked forward to not having that.
Interviewer	Tell me about having more time with each other?
Mrs. E.	Well, we go shopping together and that is a change. I would pick up the groceries after work. When we feel we want to go anywhere at any time, we just pick up and go. Like visiting. My Dad lives about 30 miles from here and he is 89 years old so we go over there quite a bit. As far as going on trips, I'm not one to travel much. We usually shared our vacation together.
Mr. E.	We go to my Army reunions. This year we are going to the company and division union. One is in July and one is in September. Now we have more time to do them things.
Mrs. E.	I would say it is just more togetherness.
Mr. E.	We go and come back when we are ready and when it suits us. If someone says stay over, we do. We had two cars before and now we are down to one.
Interviewer	Tell me about having time apart from each other, now that you are retired.
Mr. E.	I think it is good to be apart from each other every once in a while. You need time to do just as you please. If she wants to go looking for a dress, well I'm not interested in that; and if I want to shop for garden tools, she is not interested in that. It is nice to go by yourself sometimes.
Interviewer	Did you talk together about retirement before you retired?
Mr. E.	Well, she told me she was going to retire and asked me what I thought she should do and I told her it would be best if she made her own decision. I had my own retirement planned about a year ahead. I told her that I was going to retire. We all talked it over. I made my decision and she made her decision.
Mrs. E.	I may have been working longer if things would not have been the way they were at my job. The new boss took over and I did not feel like working anymore. It has been four years now since I quit and I feel good about my decision.
Interviewer	Did you talk with anyone else when you were making your decision?
Mr. E.	I talked to my supervisor and my previous supervisor. They thought it was a good decision. I had the required number of years. Most of the people who don't take it have a heart at-

tack. Someone I know who was supposed to retire the 27th of this month just had a heart attack, a bad one.

Mrs. E. I just talked to the store manager. He said whenever I wanted to quit, there would be no problem. I started to work because there is nothing to do around here. You've got to have some outlet some place and I did make a lot of friends down there. People came in to buy things and they came in regularly. You get to know them. They like me. I heard that after I left people have come into the store and asked for me. I did like working with the public. One thing about it, after I got my morning cleaning done, then you were free the rest of the day to wait on customers and talk to them. It was really a nice store to work in before we got the new boss. It was more like family. They were nice to you. The change came in the last year I worked.

Interviewer Did you have a plan for retirement?

Mr. E. My plan was after retirement, I could do as I please. If I wanted to fish or go hunting or whatever, I could do what I wanted. I could have stayed on my job til I was 70 if I wanted to and so I did not have a time set for retirement. So I did not plan that when I was 60 or 62 that I would quit. I took it year by year. I would go to meetings and every time I went, there was more paper work and more things added on. Now, I liked the work as far as being around people, but the paper work got to be too much. But I could still be working if I would have wanted to. It was too hard on my feet.

Mrs. E. Well and you also said you wanted to enjoy yourself for a while cause life is so short. You can only live one day at a time.

Mr. E. We don't have any children to worry about so we might as well enjoy ourselves. We bought a new car last year. The other was still good but we wanted a new one so we got it. Most people retire and get fat. They work hard at work and then when they retire, they get heavy.

Mrs. E. Some people get mental. They can't stand it. My Dad said that the worst thing he ever did in his life was to retire.

Mr. E. He told me. Keep on working just as long as you can. When he retired, all he did was watch television. I try to stay away from that television.

Mrs. E. Well, he did some gardening work. Just things around the house. He did not have any hobbies. I play the organ and when I feel depressed or down in the dumps, that really gives me a lift. I have had the organ for a long time. When I worked I played a little during the weekend but there really was not any time to do what you want to when you are working. Now, I have a lot of time on my hands and sometimes too much. But when I get bored I go. There is nothing to hold you back. I just get in the car and go or else take a walk.

Interviewer	Has your view of life changed since retirement?
Mr. E.	I think my view of life is better. I have no problems, no worries. We get along good. I don't have the hassle on the job. I don't have to worry about people raising heck because they raised the postage or because their letter did not get where they mailed it. This way, I don't have any worries about anything. I always had pain and gas in my lower abdomen, was always burping. Now that doesn't bother me anymore. Why I had that pain down in there for twenty years. It used to be so sore that I had to lean on a machine. Now, I don't take anything. My weight has held the same for 43 years. I still weigh 160.
Interviewer	What about your view of life, Mrs. E.?
Mrs. E.	Well, I think that after retirement, you feel closer because you're together more and do more things together. Before, we each went our separate ways. Now he's always here on time for our meals. Everything seems to go so much smoother.
Mr. E.	Before we saw each other in the morning and in the evening a little bit. Then we would each fall asleep on the Lazy Boy. Here we would each be on a Lazy Boy sleeping with the television on.
Mrs. E.	He went to work at 8 and I went to work at 9. I would get breakfast and we would hurriedly eat together. We always did get along and we talk more together about more important things.
Mr. E.	I think we do more planning now that we did before.
Mrs. E.	We do have ups and downs. Some days I just feel bored. I go for a walk or to visit my neighbors. We both like to read a lot.
Mr. E.	I'm reading more than I did before. I have more time to read and I don't fall asleep like I did when I was working. I also had a lot of reading associated with my work. Here I read my magazines and the newspapers.
Mrs. E.	I read a lot more now. Before I retired, I very seldom read anything. Now, I have different books that I am reading and I try to read the Bible every day. Before I did not have time to read the Bible at all. I'm also putting our photographs in order.
Mr. E.	I am spending more time with my brothers, too. Now, I see them every week. We just like to get together with each other.
Mrs. E.	I try to get up to see my Dad every week. I do worry about him and would like to have him here with me more, but when the weather is bad he can't get out and he was here last summer and fell. He enjoys it at my sister's place. His neighbors come and see him and he is more contented. I just wish that I lived closer so that I could help my sister and do

	more for him. He has trouble getting around, he gets short of breath.
Interviewer	What are you looking forward to?
Mr. E.	Getting out in my garden.
Mrs. E.	I want to get the house cleaned. I'm also looking forward to spring and the nice weather. Spring is my favorite season.
Mr. E.	I have two Army reunions coming up.
Interviewer	Tell me about how retirement has changed the way you talk with each other.
Mrs. E.	We have more free time and just talk more to each other.
Mr. E.	We're not as tired when we are with each other so it's just easier talking.
Mrs. E.	Right now we talk a lot about his brother, who is sick. We are concerned about him and as you get older you wonder what the future holds. I do worry about what will become of us. We will probably end up in a retirement home.
Mr. E.	I don't worry about that.
Mrs. E.	He says I worry too much. Well I do. His family is more open with things, if they have something to say, they say it and get it over with. I'm not like that. My family is not na-tured to come out and say things.
Mr. E.	We get things out in the open and off our chest and then keep on going. No grudges.
Mrs. E.	My family is more timid and keeps things more to our-selves. If something goes wrong we just keep it to ourselves. We get along good together though.
Mr. E.	Our young neighbor died suddenly and that was very hard for us. He was our closest neighbor.
Mrs. E.	She told me she would need me more now than ever and I go down to see her every day. I help her with the kids and talk to her. It was nice having a young couple so close. I de-pended on _____, because if we would have needed help, he would have been right there. But you never know, I ex-pect she will move away to be closer to her family.
Mr. E.	It was a big loss to us.
Interviewer	Since retiring what kinds of things do you see more clearly.
Mr. E.	I do think we have a lot to be thankful for and that we don't have to worry. Some people on Social Security get such lit-tle money, I don't know how they make it.
Mrs. E.	Well, I do know that I am getting older and what I thought was a little thing before now seems like a big thing. I guess the big things and the little things have switched places. Like I never watched my garden grow before. I planted it and took care of it just like I do now. But now I have time to watch it grow.

Mrs. E.	Yes, and I'm watching Jim grow. He's the neighbor's little boy and he will soon be a year old. I never had as much time to spend with a little one as I have with him.
Interviewer	What plans do you have for yourself?
Mrs. E.	I have thought about the two of us going up to the State Hospital as volunteers to help out. He is someone who can make people feel comfortable and would be good. We should look into it more.
Mr. E.	Well, you have the number, don't you?
Mrs. E.	Well, I want to take organ lessons and get a bigger organ. I have already started to look for the organ and inquire about lessons. I also want to get involved in a senior citizen center. They take trips and offer other interesting activities.
Mr. E.	I would like to do some volunteer work. We plan to look into that some more.
Interviewer	What dreams do you have for yourself?
Mr. E.	Dreams—I just hope things keep going pretty much as they are. I'm happy with the way things are.
Mrs. E.	My dream would be to move to a city closer to my Dad where there would be more to do, but when it would come time to leave, I really would not want to move. I would like to be closer to my Dad and there just isn't much to do around here. You have to drive everywhere and I would like to be someplace where you could walk or take the bus. As we get older, I don't think we will want to drive so much.

Questionnaire

1. Describe the incident of the fire at the state office building on February 5, 1981.
2. Describe your involvement in this incident.
3. Describe your reaction when you first knew that you had been exposed to a potential carcinogen.
4. How did you deal with this knowledge?
5. Describe your life before the incident.
   a. marriage
   b. relationships with other people
   c. work-interest in your job
   d. drinking, smoking habits, also drug and medication use
   e. sexuality
   f. plans for the future
   g. moods, temper
   h. sleeping patterns
6. Describe your life since the incident
   a. marriage
   b. relationships with other people
   c. work-interest in your job
   d. drinking, smoking habits, also drug and medication use
   e. sexuality
   f. plans for the future
   g. moods, temper
   h. sleeping patterns
7. Has the incident changed your life in any way?
8. Anything else you want to tell me about the situation or its meaning to you?

RESPONSES TO EACH QUESTION IN INTERVIEW GUIDE

QUESTION 1. *Describe the incident of the fire at the state office building on February 5, 1981.*

Subject 1   "You could hear what sounded like exploding—an electrical fire."

Subject 2   "There was heavy black, greasy smoke. Heavy arcing that looked like lightning. The fire in fire department terms was a five cent fire, we probably didn't use five gallons of water to extinguish it."

Subject 3   "Actually the fire itself presented no life or health hazard, but it wasn't until entering and coming back out that any of us were aware that there were PCBs."

Subject 4   "There were loud noises, lot of confusion, smoke coming out, waiting for someone to turn off the power."

Subject 5   "We couldn't see anything because the smoke was so thick. The hose felt oily, slimy and greasy. I had never encountered that before."

Subject 6   "Pretty heavy smoke, we couldn't see very far, in fact we could only feel. We were all wearing masks, the smoke left a waxy oily substance on your coat."

Subject 7   "The room was full of oily smoke, the fire was extinguished in 30 seconds."

QUESTION 2. *Describe your involvement in this situation.*

Subject 1   Subject is a union steward, he overheard the man from the electric company (who turned the power to the building off) identify the odor in the fire area as a toxic chemical.

Subject 2   Subject is assistant chief and he directed the operation.

Subject 3   Subject is a lieutenant and was first in the fire area with the captain.

Subject 4   He "went in, put it out and opened it up, ventilated it and that's it in a capsule."

Subject 5   Subject helped to extinguish the fire with the hose.

Subject 6   Subject carried portable radio, helped open door which was jammed closed.

Subject 7   Subject is the captain, went in first and relayed information back to the duty chief.

QUESTION 3.   *Describe your reaction when you first knew that you had been exposed to a potential carcinogen.*

Subject 1   "There is nothing that is ever going to be done about it and it happens all the time and nothing gets done about it."

Subject 2   That he deals with hazardous chemicals every day and "this was one more to add to the list." He stated that he was more upset because of his lack of information about the chemical and that he was "getting conflicting information from "quote experts." "I got to wondering, again, with the Nixonian attitude that we have had in this country, that maybe there is something more that I don't know about."

Subject 3   That he doesn't "overreact" but did want to know what health hazards were involved because of this exposure. He stated he has had no problems that he is aware of due to the exposure.

Subject 4   That the "doctors that we talked to were in two groups, one group tried to minimize it, the other group said it was a serious thing. I was a little bit afraid but I didn't have any reaction or rash."

Subject 5   He wasn't sure that any one really knew the nature of the exposure. He accepted the fact that he is in a dangerous profession and stated "I had no bad feelings toward it, I took every precaution that I knew how to do."

Subject 6   Doesn't like the idea that he has been exposed but accepts this. Stated, "If I don't feel any worse than I do now then I won't worry about it. If I continue to get worse, now I am going to get uptight."

Subject 7   That since he had cancer as a child and "made it through," he won't be too concerned about this incident. He stated, "You read all the time that you're exposed to carcinogenic agents in food you eat and pollutants in the air and it's just another one of those things, I suppose."

QUESTION 4.   *How did you deal with this knowledge?*

Subject 1   Since he has no signs or symptoms of liver cancer or no children with birth defects, he feels lucky. He stated, "There's no sense sitting and thinking about it on a daily basis because you outlive it or it catches up with you."

Subject 2   This specific question was not asked.

Subject 3   He doesn't give it a thought anymore.

Subject 4   "It didn't bother me much; it really didn't. I still haven't come down with cancer. There wasn't much you could do about it anyway. I really wasn't worried that much."

Subject 5   "I kind of feel that I'm a guinea pig. Either nobody knows what the danger is or they don't want to tell us. I felt though that at the first part of it they were trying to hold something back.''

Subject 6   "I don't discuss it. I don't dwell on it. You think, well maybe I have some working type thing. But you can't let it worry you, only through some instances it crops up."

Subject 7   He is in a dangerous job and that he is exposed to many toxic substances. He states, "You kind of look at it like something you can't do anything about."

QUESTION 5.   *Describe your life before the incident.*

QUESTION 6.   *Describe your life since the incident.*

All stated that there have been no changes in the specific areas questioned except Subject 5 believes he drinks more beer that he did before the incident.

QUESTION 7.   *Has the incident changed your life in any way?*

Subject 1   "The incident has made me more selfish as far as my own family goes, my personal life, my leisure time and what I want to do."

Subject 2   "When I go out that door now and I hear electrical fire I am quite concerned. Immediately PCBs pop into my mind, dioxins. I insist on full cover and minimal exposure. I've lost a lot of faith in experts."

Subject 3   "I suppose in the future if another incident occurs whereby I know there are PCBs in a confined area—well I suppose we are all going maybe to be reluctant to expose ourselves unless there is a life hazard involved."

Subject 4   There was no change but states, if they had known about it ahead of time, they could have taken standards to make sure that everyone was wearing masks.

Subject 5   "I don't take things for granted like I used to."

Subject 6   "Well, it made me think that life is a short thing and you can shorten it by being exposed. You don't know what you are going to walk into."

Subject 7   "I just don't feel that they were being honest with us. I've gotten to the point where I really appreciate life."

QUESTION 8.   *Anything else you want to tell me about the situation or its meaning to you?*

Subject 1   "Like everyone else that was there, I hope I don't suffer any long term problems from it. Not knowing, being bullshitted that was the only thing. The only thing we wanted was an answer, did something happen, do you know the answer, were we exposed?"

Subject 2   "My four score and ten is coming up pretty quick, I've got 19 years to go. If I were 23 and someone told me that this would cut your life short by 30 years, maybe 15 years down the line you are going to end up with cancer, I would be more upset than I am really."

Subject 3   "I had no ill effects and my thinking hasn't changed except I might possibly be reluctant to enter an atmosphere like that again, but if there were a life hazard involved, I'm sure it wouldn't make any difference."

Subject 4   "I still haven't come down with cancer (laugh) nobody I know has. I was affected by a rash at the time. I don't know if that was significant. I don't think it has affected me too much."

Subject 5   "I just hope that they find out if it is going to do something to us and if so, what. If they are going to find out what they are going to do about it in the years to come, if it is going to happen. I don't know if they are doing enough studies on it. But they are supposed to decide. What's 22 people out of 220 million in the United States?"

Subject 6   "I think what a person would like to say is O.K. If you have any problems and it has to do with what you were exposed to, we will take care of you. That is basically what most of us are concerned about, security, peace of mind, of being taken care of."

Subject 7   "A coverup, that is the one facet of this incident. Not the worry about what I came in contact with. I really don't think of that. The thing is the governor said he would drink a glass of the stuff. I think, what is the matter with these people that they just can't be honest with me?"

LANGUAGE PATTERNS ASSOCIATED WITH THEMES

Powering

Languaging Patterns		*Theme A. Suspicious sense of impending danger*
As subject spoke words became louder, more emphasis on each word—pitch became higher.	Subject 1	New York electric inspector could immediately identify danger inherent in coolant pyranol. "Deja vu taste" in mouth resembling agent orange experience in Vietnam Conflicting explanation of the impending danger
As subject spoke his words were slower, emphasis on many words—pitch became higher	Subject 2	Controversial opinions related to criteria signaling danger—temperature issue not resolved Child bearing spouses concerned about deformed children.
As subject spoke voice became louder, more emphasis on each word	Subject 3	Not fully aware of personal dangers of exposure to PCBs Danger signs not clearly demarcated
As subject speaks the pace of words is increased, pitch of voice is higher—a quiver is heard in his voice	Subject 4	Spouse rejects intimate contact with subject Not sure of significance of rash Laughingly states, "has not developed cancer yet"
As subject speaks—the pace of words is increased, pitch of voice is high	Subject 5	Thinks he is a "guinea pig" Either nobody knows what the danger is or "they don't want to tell us"
As subject speaks—his words are in an even, low tune	Subject 6	Concerned that he may become ill

Languaging Patterns	Theme A. Suspicious sense of impending danger	
		Worries about what may happen "five years down the road" "it's laying dormant"
As subject speaks his words are in an even, low tone	Subject 7	Not able to acquire information "When we started finding out what we had we wanted to know more about it"

	Theme B. Disillusionment with system	
As subject speaks his voice is louder, his words are faster, emphasis on each word	Subject 1	Frustration at knowing how system works No group of people is going to change until we collectively deal with the problems "Nothing ever gets done" "System inundates people with propaganda"
As subject speaks his tone is low—words are slow with emphasis on each word	Subject 2	People have attempted to get through "the system" without success Nixonion attitude pervading the system
As subject speaks—his tone is low, in an even pace	Subject 3	No one helping the firefighters on westside exposed to PCBs a week after the state office building fire
As subject speaks pitch is low, words are even tempo	Subject 4	Nothing you can do about the publicity related to the state office building fire.
As subject spoke words had more emphasis, pitch louder	Subject 5	I felt they were trying to hold something back Felt something could be done before
As subject spoke his tone was low, there are pauses between thoughts and phrases—emphasis on words	Subject 6	They should have been more open with us instead of reading it in the newspaper Made us feel that the building is of more concern than the people involved basically I am just a number and I will be for years State has immunity, can absolve themselves Almost as if the governor had no feeling toward us.

Languaging Patterns	Theme B.	*Disillusionment with system*
As subject spoke his tone and pitch of voice became higher, louder	Subject 7	Information came very slowly from the Health Department, almost as if they were putting us off We were being lied to—the state tried to play this down
	Theme C.	*Explicit and implicit reference to mortality*
As subject spoke his tone was low, emphasis on each word, tone became higher	Subject 1	Unable to document PCB blood level since samples were lost Hoping medical science will develop "bionic man" to deal with mortality
As subject spoke his tone and pitch of voice became higher—more emphasis on words	Subject 2	No known cure for dioxin poison—"Make your will" No one has done a biopsy to determine actual presence of PCBs, that's the only way you *really* know.
As subject spoke his tone and pitch of voice were low, even	Subject 3	Concern over health—wants to be around 30–40 years "if possible" No one could enter the state office building and "live"
As subject spoke voice had high pitch, a quiver is heard in his voice	Subject 4	"Life could end abruptly" Cancer and asbestos cause death
As subject spoke his tone and pitch were low—words spoken at the same rate	Subject 5	Hopes to stay in good health, if they ever find anything that can be done for these exposed to "prevent something some how" Not afraid of dying—doesn't want to die of cancer
As subject spoke his voice was low-pitched, rate slow—hesitant	Subject 6	"You are playing a game and just waiting" Life is short and you can shorten it by being exposed to things You feel what a waste if it takes your life
As subject spoke his words were low, tone low	Subject 7	The value of life reinforced coming in contact with a substance that could shorten it

Languaging Patterns	*Theme D. Distrust of experts*	
As subject spoke his voice was low—emphasis on each word—tempo slow	Subject 1	Conflicting medical opinions related to severity of exposure. Not "officially" notified of test results
As subject spoke his words were slow, emphasis on each word—tempo and tone low	Subject 2	Conflicting information from the "quote experts" "Loss of faith" in experts Professionals telling subject to choose up sides relating to technical information
As subject spoke the tempo was slow, voice low	Subject 3	People responded to "overreaction by state building experts"
As subject spoke the tempo was fast, tone high	Subject 4	Medical experts disagreed on seriousness of health hazard. Conflicting opinions about when blood tests should be done
As subject spoke his sentences were rapid, tone high	Subject 5	Nobody really knows—if they do they're not saying "I don't know if they've done enough studies on it" "They took the situation lightly"
As subject spoke his tone was low, emphasis on each word—tempo slow	Subject 6	"Wonder how much Monsanto who made the pyranol tested this under heat—did they know it produced these other things" "Newspapers and professors saying how toxic dioxins are and then having sensationalized it in the newspapers."
As subject spoke tempo slower and tone lower.	Subject 7	"Experts said blood tests, then became vague with us—blood frozen, thawed—inconclusive."

LANGUAGING PATTERNS ASSOCIATED WITH CHOICES FOR THE FUTURE

Enabling—Limiting

Languaging Patterns		*Choices related to the future*
As the subject spoke each word was emphatically pronounced—the tone was low, tempo slow	Subject 1	Subject chooses to remain with firefighting company and accepts risks related to job. He believes he is more caring with his family since the incident but not sure if it is related to the incident per se. He hopes he won't suffer long-term problems from the incident in the future. "Yes, I am more caring about my family." "I don't think it's the state office building incident—we are closer now." "I hope I don't suffer any long-term problems from it."
As subject spoke his voice was low, tempo slow	Subject 2	Subject chooses to remain with firefighting company and accepts the risks related to the job. He believes that the family accepts the dangers. He believes that he will live to old age "gracefully." "I love my profession and I'm very happy in it." "Family knows danger—have been to funeral of other firefighters." "I figure on staying around here for another 10 or 11 years, God willing and then

Languaging Patterns		*Choices related to the future*
		take my normal retirement and go into old age very, very gracefully."
As subject spoke the tone of voice was low, tempo slow	Subject 3	Subject chooses to remain with firefighting company. He believes wife is not concerned—at least she doesn't show it. Though he believes he isn't in danger he says he might be reluctant to enter an atmosphere like that again. "My wife is not concerned— at least not outwardly. I can't tell whether she's concerned or not." "I don't feel I'm in any danger." "I might possibly be reluctant to enter an atmosphere like that again."
As subject spoke his voice quivered, tone low, tempo fast	Subject 4	Subject chooses to remain with firefighting company and accepts risks related to job. Postponed decision to have children—may not or may be related to incident. He expects to go along the way he is until retirement and then travel. Indecisive about having children. "Health hazards are part of the job." Plans to go along the way he is now.
As subject spoke the tone of voice had a high pitch quality, tempo fast	Subject 5	Subject plans to remain with firefighting company even though he knows there are dangers inherent in the job. He is more careful when responding to a call now because he worries about another similar incident. He plans to retire after 20 years. "I didn't really have any bad feelings" "I knew the job had dangerous aspects or I wouldn't be here"

Languaging Patterns		*Choices related to the future*
		"I don't take chances" "I worry about another incident" "I don't take things for granted like I used to."
As subject spoke his tone of voice was low, tempo slow	Subject 6	Subject is 52 years old and looks forward to retiring at 55. He states that this is a young man's job. Does have plans for retirement and is buying mountain property. Feels that if there was another problem none of the people would hesitate to handle it. Wants to fish and do carpentry. Buying mountain property. "No reason why I can't" (about retirement) "I think none of the people would hesitate to handle it the way they should."
As subject spoke his tone of voice was low, tempo slow	Subject 7	Subject feels dangers are inherent in his job and is something that can't be changed. He had cancer as a child and feels that he appreciates life. He is saving and planning for the future. "It is the type of job we have" "Like something you can't do anything about" "I have gotten to the point where I really appreciate life" "I want to put our kids through college and retire with financial security."

EPILOGUE

This text is the first nursing research book to set forth selected qualitative methods within a nursing perspective, including demonstration chapters reporting completed research. One nursing perspective was used with all of the methods to demonstrate the internal consistency required within the rigorous processes of qualitative research. The nursing perspective used in this work, the theory of Man-Living-Health, is written in abstruse language consistent with the nature of theory in scientific disciplines. Learning the theory in scientific disciplines requires formal study, a reverence for quiet contemplation, and creative synthesis. Neither the theory nor the methodologies presented in this work can be learned quickly. The nature of the content compels the learner to abide with the conceptualizations and study the movements in discourse required by scholars who aspire to contribute to research and theory development in nursing.

The results of the major studies in this work demonstrate comparable findings which complement each other and support the theory of Man-Living-Health. Meaning, rhythmicity, and transcendence, the three major themes, which surface from the assumptions and give rise to the three principles of Man-Living-Health, can be seen in varying ways in all studies. All three themes emerged in the common elements of the phenomenological study describing health for 400 subjects in four age groups. The common elements of plentitude, harmony, and energy for all groups demonstrated a clear shift in focus for each of the four groups. The shift in focus was from an intense immersion in movement and struggle for younger subjects, toward a more contemplative engagement with purposefulness and significant completion for older subjects.

The phenomenological study of *Persisting in Change* revealed some similarities with the middle adult groups in the health study, in that the subjects struggled with the certainty-uncertainty of initiating new projects in light of reordering interrelational connections. There was considerable turbulence in the changes described; hence the immersion in movement and struggle.

In the exploratory study related to the meaning of being exposed to toxic chemicals, the movement and struggle are seen in the deliberate choice to stay with the risk of known present dangers and questionable future consequences. The immersion in this struggle for the firefighters focused the meaning of their interrelationships on a profound re-evaluation of value priorities.

Contemplative engagement with purposefulness and significant completions was most evident in the fourth group of the health study, and coincides with the results of the ethnographic and case studies, both of which investigated older adults. In the ethnographic study, this contemplative engagement was seen in the quiet struggle of the old to make livable the concrete realities of their changing worlds. The new awarenesses of self-as-old were made explicit through changes in patterns of interrelating and through the dawning realization of personal non-being. These new awarenesses generated remembrances of the past as they transformed the present in the struggle to give meaning to an increasingly unsure and limited future.

In the case study, contemplative engagement was seen as the retired couple struggled with the decision to retire or continue working, and in the subsequent satisfaction experienced after retiring. The changing pattern of their lives, freely embraced in retirement, generated new possibilities for more meaningful relationships, more satisfying individual projects, and freedom to structure time in a more flexible way.

In all studies, then, shifting rhythms of connecting-separating surfaced as subjects originated creative ways of transforming life patterns in light of changing valued images and reordered priorities. This conclusion gives evidence of support for the theory of Man-Living-Health, and demonstrates the logical consistency present when using a variety of qualitative methods of inquiry with one nursing perspective.

Setting forth a logically congruent text, though always verbally sought, is considered by some to be a dangerous endeavor. It posits yet another standard by which to judge the emergence of nursing as a scientific discipline. Where there is danger, however, there is also opportunity. Setting and living a standard in a discipline calls forth a strong undercurrent of conflict to temper the rapid movement of the standard as a new wave. The undercurrent is an example of the pushing-resisting paradox; while seemingly a resistant force, it acts to shift the sands and push the wave to greater heights. And so it is, in the pushing-resisting rhythm of scholarly dialogue about a work, that conflict surfaces and shifts the views in the ongoing emergence of nursing as a scientific discipline.

GLOSSARY

BRACKETING Suspending belief in the existence of a phenomenon through parenthetical inclusion.

COCONSTITUTION Man's active participation in creating meaning with others in the world.*

COEXISTENCE Living with predecessors, contemporaries and successors all at once.*

DESCRIPTIVE METHOD A qualitative method of inquiry directed toward providing meaningful and accurate explorations of the background and environmental interactions of a given social event.

EMIC APPROACH The insider's view as expressed in the language of a given culture.

ETHNOGRAPHIC INQUIRY Complex way of interrelating with informants that includes appropriately informal conversation and deliberate, focused questioning designed to elicit rich cultural meanings.

ETHNOGRAPHIC METHOD A qualitative method of inquiry directed toward learning the meaning of experience through the cultural perspective of the group being studied.

ETIC APPROACH The outsider's view of the occurrence of events as described by the researcher.

GENERAL INFORMANT An informal participant in part of an ethnographic study.

INTERSUBJECTIVITY Subject-subject relationship involving a true presence.*

KEY INFORMANT A consistent participant throughout an ethnographic study.

LANGUAGING Sharing valued images through symbols, words, gesture, gaze, touch and posture.*

*Rosemarie Rizzo Parse, *Man-Living-Health: A Theory of Nursing* (New York: John Wiley & Sons, 1981).

LIVING UNITY   An experiencing subject who is more than and different from the sum of parts.*

MAN-LIVING-HEALTH   A unitary phenomenon referring to Man's becoming through cocreating rhythmical patterns of relating while cotranscending in open interchange with the environment.*

NEGENTROPY   Process of evolving toward greater complexity and diversity.

PARADIGM   A way of viewing a particular phenomenon.

PARTICIPANT OBSERVATIONS   A way of involved watching.

PHENOMENOLOGICAL ANALYSIS   A rigorous process of intuiting, analyzing, and describing the tacit and explicit meaning of experiences presented by subjects.

PHENOMENOLOGICAL METHOD   A qualitative method of inquiry directed toward uncovering the meaning of human experience from the perspective of the experiencing person.

QUALITATIVE RESEARCH   An approach to inquiry that yields descriptive characteristics.

QUANTITATIVE RESEARCH   An approach to inquiry that yields numerical indicators.

RESEARCH PROCESS   The scientific exploration of phenomenon through examination of conceptual, ethical, methodological and interpretative dimensions.

SYNERGISTIC   Mutually and simultaneously enhancing.*

TRANSCENDING   Going beyond; exceeding.*

BIBLIOGRAPHY

Aamodt, Agnes. "Examining Ethnography for Nurse Researchers." *Western Journal of Nursing Research*, 4:209–221, 1982.

Aamodt, Agnes M. "Problems in Doing Nursing Research: Developing a Criteria for Evaluating Qualitative Research." *Western Journal of Nursing Research*, 5:398–402, 1983.

Batey, Marjorie V. "Conceptualization: Knowledge and Logic Guiding the Research Process." *Nursing Research*, 26:324–329, 1977.

Becker, H., et al. *Boys in White*. Chicago: The University of Chicago Press, 1961.

Bodgan, Robert and Stephen J. Taylor. *Introduction to Qualitative Research Methods*. New York: John Wiley & Sons, 1975.

Brody, Howard and Daniel S. Sobel. "A Systems View of Health and Disease" in *Ways of Health*. D. S. Sobel, ed. New York: Harcourt, Brace, Jovanovich. 1979.

Buber, Martin. *The Knowledge of Man*. New York: Harper and Row, 1965.

Campbell, D. T. "The informant in qualitative research." *American Journal of Sociology*. Chicago: Rand McNally, 1966.

Clement, Imelda W. and Florence B. Roberts, eds. *Family Health: a Theoretical Approach to Nursing Care*. New York: John Wiley & Sons, 1983.

Colby, Benjamin. "Culture Grammars." *Science*, 187:4180, 1975.

de Beauvoir, Simeone. *The Coming of Age*. New York: Warner Books, Inc., 1973.

Dilthey, Wilhem. *Pattern and Meaning in History*. New York: Harper & Row, 1961.

Donaldson, S. K. and D. M. Crowley. "The Disciplines of Nursing." *Nursing Outlook*, 26:113–120, 1978.

Erikson, Eric. *Childhood and Society*. New York: W. W. Norton and Co., Inc., 1963.

Evameshko, Margarita and Kay Artschwager. "Ethnoscience Research Technique." *Western Journal of Nursing Research*, 4:49–64, 1982.

Fabrega, H. "The Need for an Ethnomedical Science." *Science*, 189:935–969, 1975.

Febrega, H. "The Ethnography of Illness." *Social Science and Medicine*. 1979. 13:565–76.

Fawcett, Jacqueline. *Analysis and Evaluation of Conceptual Models of Nursing*. Philadelphia: F. A. Davis Company, 1984.

Filstead, W., ed. *Qualitative Methodology: Firsthand Involvement with the Social World*. Chicago: Markham, 1970.

Frake, Charles O. *Structural Descriptions of Sunbanum Religious Behavior*, Ward Goodenough, ed. New York: McGraw-Hill, 1964.

Frankl, Victor E. "Significance of the Meaning of Health." in *Religion and*

Medicine. by D. R. Belgum, pp. 177–185. Iowa: Iowa State University Press, 1967.

Giorgi, Amedeo. *Psychology as a Human Science.* New York: Harper and Row, 1970.

Giorgi, Amedeo, William F. Fisher, and Rolf Von Eckartsberg. *Duquesne Studies in Phenomenological Psychology.* Vol. 1. Pittsburgh: Duquesne University Press, 1971.

Giorgi, Amedeo, Constance T. Fischer, and Edward L. Murray, eds., Convergence and Divergence of Qualitative and Quantitative Methods of Psychology, in *Phenomenological Psychology*, Vol. 2, Pittsburgh: Duquesne University Press, 1975.

Giorgi, Amedeo, C. L. Fischer, and E. L. Murray. *Duquesne Studies in Phenomenological Psychology*: Pittsburgh: Duquesne University Press, 1975.

Glaser, Barney G. and Anselm L. Strauss. *The Discovery of Grounded Theory: Strategies for Qualitative Research.* New York: Aldine Publishing Co., 1967.

Gorenberg, Bobby E., "The Research Tradition of Nursing: An Emerging Issue." *Nursing Research*, 32:347–349, 1983.

Harris, Marvin. "Why a Perfect Knowledge of All the Rules One Must Know to Act Like a Native Cannot Lead to the Knowledge of How Natives Act." *Journal of Anthropological Research*. 30:242–251. 1974.

Harris, Marvin. *The Rise of Anthropological Theory.* New York: Thomas Y. Crowell Co., Inc. 1968.

Heidegger, Martin. *Being and Time.* New York: Harper and Row, 1962.

Human Guidelines for Nurses in Clinical and Other Research. American Nurses Association, 1975.

Isaac, Stephen and William B. Michael, *Handbook in Research and Evaluation.* San Diego: Edits Publishers, 1981.

Jacobs, G., ed. *The Participant Observer.* New York: Braziller, 1970.

Jacobs, J. "A Phenomenological Study of Suicide Notes." *Social Problems*, 15 (Summer):60–72, 1967.

Kaplan, Abraham. *The Conduct of Inquiry: Methodology for Behavioral Science.* Scranton, Pennsylvania: Chandler Publishing Company, 1964.

Katchadourian, Herant. *Medical Perspectives on Adulthood.* in Erik Erikson ed. Adulthood. New York: W. W. Norton Co., Inc., 1978.

Kempler, Walter. *Principles of Gestalt Family Therapy*, Salt Lake City: Deseret Press, 1974.

Knaack, Phyllis. "Phenomenological Research," *Western Journal of Nursing Research*, 6:107–114, 1984.

Knafl, Kathleen Astin and Marion J. Howard. "Interpreting and Reporting Qualitative Research." *Research in Nursing and Health*, 7:17–24, 1984.

Kuhn, Thomas. *The Structure of Scientific Revolutions.* Chicago: University of Chicago Press, 1970.

Lauden, Larry. *Progress and Its Problems.* Berkeley, California: University of California Press, 1977.

Leininger, Madeline. "Introduction: Nature of Science in Nursing." *Nursing Research*, 18:388–389, 1969.

Leininger, M. *Nursing and Anthropology: Two Worlds to Blend.* New York: John Wiley & Sons, 1970.

Lofland, J. "Editorial Introduction—Analyzing Qualitative Data: First Person Accounts." *Urban Life and Culture*, 3 (October):307–309, 1974.

Lofland, J. "Styles of reporting qualitative field research." *The American Sociologist*, 8 (August):101–111, 1974.

Luijpen, William A. *Existential Phenomenology*. New York: Humanities Press, 1960.

Marcel, Gabriel. *The Philosophy of Existentialism*. Secaucus, New Jersey: The Citadel Press, 1956.

Mayeroff, Milton. *On Caring*. New York: Harper and Row, 1971.

Merleau-Ponty, Maurice, (translated by Colin Smith). *Phenomenology of Perception*. New York: Humanities Press, 1974.

Neugarten, Bernice, ed. *Middle Age and Aging*. Chicago: The University of Chicago Press, 1968.

Newman, Margaret. *Theory Development in Nursing*. Philadelphia: F. A. Davis, 1979.

Oiler, Carolyn. "The Phenomenological Approach in Nursing Research." *Nursing Research*, 31:178–181, 1982.

Omery, Anna. "Phenomenology: A Method for Nursing Research." 5:49–63, 1983.

Parse, Rosemarie Rizzo. *Man-Living-Health: A Theory of Nursing*. New York: John Wiley & Sons, 1981.

Pelto, Pertti J. and Gretel H. Pelto. *Anthropological Research: The Structure of Inquiry*. Cambridge: Cambridge University Press. 1981.

Phillips, Bernard. *Social Research Strategy and Tactics*. New York: MacMillan, 1972.

Polit, D. and D. Hungler, *Nursing Research: Principles and Method*. Philadelphia: J. B. Lippincott Co., 1983.

Ragucci, Antoinette T. "The Ethnographic Approach and Nursing Research." *Nursing Research*, 21:485–490, 1972.

Raths, Louis E., Merrill Harmin, and Sidney B. Simon. *Values and Teaching: Working with Volumes in the Classroom*. Columbia, Ohio: Charles E. Merrill, 1978.

Riehl, Joan P. and Callista Roy. *Conceptual Models for Nursing Practice*. New York: Appleton-Century-Crofts, 1980.

Rogers, Martha E. *An Introduction to the Theoretical Basis of Nursing*. Philadelphia: F. A. Davis, 1970.

Rosenhan, D. L. "On Being Sane in Insane Places." *Science*, 179 (4070) (January):250–258, 1973.

Roy, Callista and Sharon L. Roberts. *Theory Construction in Nursing: An Adaptation Model*. Englewood Cliffs, New Jersey: Prentice-Hall, Inc., 1981.

Roy, Callista. *Introduction to Nursing: An Adaption Model*. (2nd Edition). Englewood Cliffs, New Jersey: Prentice-Hall, Inc., 1984.

Sartre, Jean-Paul. *Being and Nothingness*. New York: Washington Square Press. 1966.

Saunders, William B. and Thomas K. Pinkey. *The Conduct of Social Research*. New York: Holt, Rinehart and Winston, 1983.

Segall, M. *Human Behavior in Cross-Cultural Psychology: Global Perspective*. Monterey, CA: Brooks/Cole, 1979.

Shaw, C. R. "Case study method." *Publications of The American Sociological Society*, 21:149–157, 1927.

Spiegelberg, Herbert. *The Phenomenological Movement*. Vols. I and II. The Hague: Martinus Nijhoff, 1976.

Spradley, James P. *Participant Observation*. New York: Holt, Rinehart and Winston, 1980.

_____. *The Ethnographic Interview*. New York: Holt, Rinehart and Winston, 1979.

Sturtevant, William C. "Studies in Ethnoscience." in *Theory in Anthropology*. R. Manners and D. Kaplan, eds. Chicago: Aldine-Atherton Press, 1968.

Strasser, Stephan. *Phenomenology and the Human Sciences*. Pittsburgh: Duquesne University Press, 1963.

Swanson, Janice and Carole Chenits. Why Qualitative Research in Nursing? *Nursing Outlook*, 30:241–245, 1982.

Tillich, Paul. *Love, Power and Justice*. New York: Oxford University Press, 1954.

Tiryakian, E. "Existential Phenomenology and Sociology." *American Sociological Review*, 30 (October):674–688, 1965.

Trow, M. "Comment on 'Participant Observation and Interviewing a Comparison.' " *Human Organization*, 16(3):33–35, 1957.

Truzzi, M., ed. *Subjective Understanding in the Social Sciences*. Reading, Massachusetts: Addison-Wesley, 1974.

Turner, R., ed. *Ethnomethodology*. Baltimore: Penguin, 1974.

vanKaam, Adrian. *Existential Foundations of Psychology*. New York: Doubleday, 1969.

_____. *Living Creatively*. Denville, Dimension Books, 1972.

Vidich, A. J. & Bensman, J. "The Validity of Field Data." *Human Organization*, 13(1):20–27, 1954.

Watson, Jean. "Nursing's Scientific Quest," *Nursing Outlook*, 29:413–416, 1981.

Werner, O. "Structural Anthropology" in *Main Currents in Cultural Anthropology*. R. Naroll and F. Naroll, eds. Englewood Cliffs, NJ: Prentice-Hall, 1973.

Zelditch, M., Jr. "Some Methodological Problems of Field Studies." *American Journal of Sociology*, 67:566–675, 1962.

INDEX